Register Now for Online Access to Your Bo

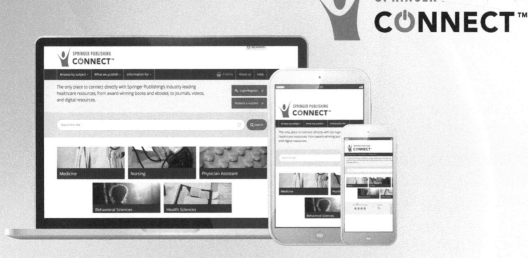

Your print purchase of *Medical Imaging for the Health Care Provider: Practical Radiograph Interpretation, Second Edition,* **includes online access to the contents of your book**—increasing accessibility, portability, and searchability!

Access today at:
http://connect.springerpub.com/content/book/978-0-8261-6047-8
or scan the QR code at the right with your smartphone. Log in or register, then click "Redeem a voucher" and use the code below.

> **SEUFFKA0**

Scan here for quick access.

Having trouble redeeming a voucher code?
Go to https://connect.springerpub.com/redeeming-voucher-code

If you are experiencing problems accessing the digital component of this product, please contact our customer service department at cs@springerpub.com

The online access with your print purchase is available at the publisher's discretion and may be removed at any time without notice.

Publisher's Note: New and used products purchased from third-party sellers are not guaranteed for quality, authenticity, or access to any included digital components.

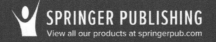

SPRINGER PUBLISHING
View all our products at springerpub.com

SPC

Medical Imaging for the Health Care Provider

Theresa M. Campo, DNP, FNP-C, FAANP, FAAN, is the Vice President of Accreditation, Conference, and Education for the American Association of Nurse Practitioners. Dr. Campo was chair of the department of EMS and Director for the Emergency Nurse Practitioner track at Drexel University. She is board certified as a family nurse practitioner with licensure in multiple states. She has over 30 years of experience in the emergency setting, including prehospital, emergency department/quick care, and trauma. Dr. Campo is an inaugural fellow of the Coldiron Senior Executive Fellowship and received her doctor of nursing practice from Case Western Reserve University, Cleveland, Ohio, and her master of science in nursing, family nurse practitioner, from Widener University, Chester, Pennsylvania. She is a national and international lecturer on emergency and urgent care topics. In addition to *Medical Imaging for the Health Care Provider*, Dr. Campo is the co-editor of *Essential Procedures for the Emergency, Urgent, and Primary Care Settings: A Clinical Companion, Third Edition*, and *Emergency Nurse Practitioner Core Curriculum*, and has authored several book chapters and peer-reviewed articles. Dr. Campo was awarded the American Association of Nurse Practitioners (AANP) State Award for Excellence in 2011 and was inducted into the fellows of the AANP (FAANP) in 2015. She is also a fellow of the American Academy of Nursing (FAAN) since 2017.

Medical Imaging for the Health Care Provider

Practical Radiograph Interpretation

Second Edition

THERESA M. CAMPO, DNP, FNP-C, FAANP, FAAN

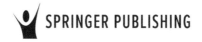 SPRINGER PUBLISHING

First Springer Publishing edition 2017, 978-0-8261-3126-3.

Springer Publishing Company, LLC
www.springerpub.com
connect.springerpub.com

Executive Acquisitions Editor: Joseph Morita
Director, Content Development: Taylor Ball
Production Editor: Kris Parrish
Compositor: Amnet

ISBN: 978-0-8261-6046-1
ebook ISBN: 978-0-8261-6047-8
DOI: 10.1891/9780826160478

SUPPLEMENTS:
Instructor Materials:
Image Bank ISBN: 978-0-8261-6048-5

Qualified instructors may request supplements by emailing textbook@springerpub.com

Video Transcripts ISBN: 978-0-8261-6049-2

23 24 25 26 / 5 4 3 2 1

The author and the publisher of this Work have made every effort to use sources believed to be reliable to provide information that is accurate and compatible with the standards generally accepted at the time of publication. Because medical science is continually advancing, our knowledge base continues to expand. Therefore, as new information becomes available, changes in procedures become necessary. We recommend that the reader always consult current research and specific institutional policies before performing any clinical procedure or delivering any medication. The author and publisher shall not be liable for any special, consequential, or exemplary damages resulting, in whole or in part, from the readers' use of, or reliance on, the information contained in this book. The publisher has no responsibility for the persistence or accuracy of URLs for external or third-party Internet websites referred to in this publication and does not guarantee that any content on such websites is, or will remain, accurate or appropriate.

Library of Congress Cataloging-in-Publication Data

Names: Campo, Theresa M., author.
Title: Medical imaging for the health care provider : practical radiograph interpretation / Theresa M. Campo.
Description: Second edition. | New York : Springer Publishing Company, [2024] | Includes bibliographical references and index.
Identifiers: LCCN 2023013429 (print) | LCCN 2023013430 (ebook) | ISBN 9780826160461 (paperback) | ISBN 9780826160478 (ebook)
Subjects: MESH: Diagnostic Imaging--methods | Image Interpretation, Computer-Assisted--methods
Classification: LCC RC78.7.D53 (print) | LCC RC78.7.D53 (ebook) | NLM WN 180 | DDC 616.07/54--dc23/eng/20230605
LC record available at https://lccn.loc.gov/2023013429
LC ebook record available at https://lccn.loc.gov/2023013430

Contact sales@springerpub.com to receive discount rates on bulk purchases.

Publisher's Note: **New and used products purchased from third-party sellers are not guaranteed for quality, authenticity, or access to any included digital components.**

Printed in the United States of America by Gasch Printing.

I dedicate this book to my husband Jonathan. You never cease to amaze me with your support, encouragement, guidance, and, most of all, love. This book would not have come to fruition without you! You are the reason I wake up in the morning, you are the love of my life, and you are my best friend and soul mate. God certainly blessed me with you.

CONTENTS

REVIEWERS

David Angelastro, MD, FACEP Director, Emergency Medicine, Bayfront Emergency Physicians, Shore Memorial Hospital, Somers Point, New Jersey

David Begleiter, MD Clinical Managing Member, Atlantic Medical Imaging, Galloway, New Jersey

Kathleen Bradbury-Golas, DNP, RN, FNP-C, ACNS-BC Associate Clinical Professor in Graduate Nursing, Nurse Practitioner, MSN Department, College of Nursing and Health Professions, Drexel University, Philadelphia, Pennsylvania

Kyle Deuter, PA-C Certified Physician Assistant, Bone and Joint Institute of South Georgia, Jesup, Georgia

Dian Dowling Evans, PhD, FNP-BC, ENP-BC, FAANP Associate Professor and Director of the Family/Emergency Nurse Practitioner Program, Emory University, Atlanta, Georgia; Emergency Nurse Practitioner, Emory University Hospital and Emory Midtown Emergency Departments, Atlanta, Georgia

Johnny S. Gomes, DO, AAEM Emergency Medicine Specialist, Frye Regional Medical Center, Hickory, North Carolina; Functional and Integrative Medicine, Physician, Director, Optimal Healthcare and Wellness PLLC, Morganton, North Carolina

Anne Hedger, DNP, ACNP-BC, ANP-BC, CPNP-AC, ENP-BC Emergency Nurse Practitioner, Providence Newberg Medical Center; Acute Care Pediatric Nurse Practitioner Program Coordinator, University of South Alabama, Mobile, Alabama

Boris Libster, DO Allied Gastrointestinal Associates, P.A., Haddon Heights and Voorhies, New Jersey

Todd Luyber, DO, FAAEM Atlantic Emergency Associates, AtlantiCare Regional Medical Center, Atlantic City, New Jersey

David G. MacBride, DO, CPE, FACEP Medical Director, AtlantiCare Regional Medical Center, Pomona, New Jersey

Yatish B. Merchant, MD, FACC, MBBS AtlantiCare Physician Group, Galloway, New Jersey

Aubrey Rybyinski, BS, RDMS, RVT Lead Technologist, Navix Diagnostix, Taunton, Massachusetts

William Schumacher, DO, FACEP EMS Director, Bayfront Emergency Physicians, Shore Memorial Hospital, Somers Point, New Jersey

Allen Lewis Silvey Jr., DO Pulmonary/Critical Care Medicine, MedCorps Asthma and Pulmonary Specialists, Turnersville, New Jersey

LIST OF SUPPLEMENTARY VIDEOS

Please visit https://connect.springerpub.com/content/book/978-0-8261-6047-8/chapter /ch00 to access the videos.

▶ VIDEOS

Ch 4: Basic Interpretation of the Chest

4.1: Introduction

4.2: Interpretation of the Chest—Normal

Ch 5: Abnormalities Found on Radiographs of the Chest

5.1: Interpretation of the Chest—Density Abnormalities

5.2: Interpretation of the Chest—Air Abnormalities

Ch 6: Basic Interpretation of Radiographs of the Abdomen

6.1: Interpretation of the Abdomen—Normal

6.2: Interpretation of the Abdomen—Free Air

6.3: Interpretation of the Abdomen—Small and Large Bowel Abnormalities

Ch 7: Basic Interpretation of Long Bone—Upper Extremity Radiographs

7.1: Interpretation—Extremity

7.2: Interpretation—Normal Shoulder, Humerus, and Clavicle

7.3: Interpretation—Humeral Head Fracture

7.4: Interpretation—Normal Elbow, Radius, and Ulna

7.5: Interpretation—Radial Head Fracture

7.6: Interpretation—Collies Fracture

7.7: Interpretation—Boxer's Fracture

7.8: Interpretation—Finger Fracture

FOREWORD TO THE FIRST EDITION

When medical professionals are confronted with interpreting their own patients' x-ray studies, the task can seem daunting. In her new book, *Medical Imaging for the Health Care Provider: Practical Radiograph Interpretation*, Dr. Theresa Campo reduces the seemingly overwhelming task into manageable, logical steps. She literally takes you through the ABCs of interpretation. The information is relevant, practical, and immediately applicable to the modern medical provider.

If that weren't enough, Dr. Campo also is able to provide insight into the sometimes-confusing alphabet soup of imaging, giving real-world guidance in how and when to order an ultrasound, MRI, and CT. By expertly explaining the hows and whys of imaging, she provides you with a powerful tool for understanding what to order for your patient, rather than reverting to a laundry list that you can never remember or that never seems to exactly be applicable to the situation you are in.

These insights, along with a thorough knowledge of relevant terms and vocabulary that is so necessary in communication among medical professionals, makes this book one you will want to have by your side every day you are working. I know you'll enjoy and appreciate *Medical Imaging for the Health Care Provider*.

David Begleiter, MD
Clinical Managing Member
Atlantic Medical Imaging
Galloway, New Jersey

PREFACE

Welcome to *Medical Imaging for the Health Care Provider: Practical Radiograph Interpretation.* I prepared this book after I discovered a lack of suitable resources when teaching classes to nurse practitioner students in medical imaging and interpretation. I simply wanted to share the excitement I have for this topic with my advanced practice, interdisciplinary colleagues and help them understand the dynamics of the five testing modalities and approaches to interpretation of radiographs. I truly believe this book can be useful to all health care providers, whether students or practicing providers, in a wide range of clinical settings.

The intention of this book is to provide a concise, easy-to-use reference that introduces the reader to differences in medical imaging testing modalities and teaches the basics of plain radiograph interpretation. It is designed to assist providers in identifying and understanding the various medical imaging testing modalities of radiographs, CTs, nuclear imaging, MRIs, and ultrasound scans and images. The book presents written descriptions of the various modalities that are enhanced with figures, tables, and actual patient films. The text demonstrates concepts and discusses in clearly presented language the various attributes of the range of testing modalities and how to interpret them. This approach helps to deepen the practitioner's understanding of the differences in the modalities, along with a deeper appreciation for the parameters of these tests and supports appropriate utilization of these diagnostic tools when diagnosing patients.

This book is divided into four units. The first unit introduces the reader to the history of medical imaging and gives an overview of radiology and each testing modality. Guidance is provided on how to choose the best diagnostic medical imaging test to assess the presenting condition. Units II through IV cover interpretation of plain radiographs of the chest, abdomen, extremities, and spine. Age-appropriate considerations are included throughout the book, as is the importance of the clinical decision-making process. To enhance learning, this edition includes a collection of 30 narrated videos that provide thorough, step-by-step guidance on x-ray interpretation for normal and abnormal findings. **The reader may also access the videos found in this text at** http://connect.springerpub.com/content /book/978-0-8261-6047-8/chapter/ch00.

Interpretation of plain radiographs can be challenging and frustrating for any provider, whether student or novice. The simplified approach to interpretation is performed step by step utilizing the ABCs of interpretation. Having fail-safe measures in place, learning to interpret what you are seeing on the radiograph, and understanding the rationale underlying your interpretation will assist you in confidently diagnosing the patient. Whether you are reading a radiology report or interpreting radiographs, this important resource will help build your confidence in your ability to read and interpret radiographs. It will help you feel more self-assured and less stressed. So, let's get started and have fun!

Theresa M. Campo

ACKNOWLEDGMENTS

One person cannot move mountains or accomplish goals by themselves. My family, friends, and colleagues have helped me to accomplish my goal of publishing this book. I would like to say thank you for your continued support!

Dad, I want to thank you for the unconditional support you give me. You mean the world to me, and I am so blessed with the relationship we have grown into. You are not only my father but a person I look up to and admire.

Atlantic Medical Imaging—radiology group—thank you for all your support and guidance in developing and completing this book. Dr. David Begleiter, especially—thank you for all your guidance, expertise, support, encouragement, and most of all the patience you gave me during the journey in completing this book.

Joe Morita and Springer Publishing Company—thank you for allowing me the opportunity to share my love for medical imaging with my colleagues.

I would like to thank the following individuals for assisting with illustrations and images. You were more than instrumental in making this book complete.

David Begleiter, MD
Clinical Managing Member
Atlantic Medical Imaging
Galloway, New Jersey

Douglas W. Parrillo, MD
Chairman, Department of Radiological Sciences
Drexel University College of Medicine
Clinical Service Chief of Radiology
Hahnemann University Hospital, Tenethealth
Philadelphia, Pennsylvania

Kyle Deuter, PA-C
Certified Physician Assistant
Bone and Joint Institute of South Georgia
Jesup, Georgia

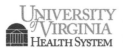

UNIVERSITY *of* VIRGINIA HEALTH SYSTEM | Department of Radiology & Medical Imaging

I would like to thank Heather Cox and the students from Ocean City High School who provided the awesome drawings for this book.

Heather Cox
Art Teacher
Ocean City High School
Ocean City, New Jersey

Illustrators
John Brittin Jr.
Jack Crowell
Matt Colbert
Andrew Haines
Paul Kenney
David Rosario

SPRINGER PUBLISHING CONNECT™ RESOURCES

Resources designed to supplement this text are located at http://connect.springerpub
.com/content/book/978-0-8261-6047-8/chapter/ch00

- Supplementary Videos are available to all purchasers of this text. See List of
  Supplementary Videos for detailed information.

- An Image Bank is available to qualified instructors by emailing textbook@springerpub
  .com.

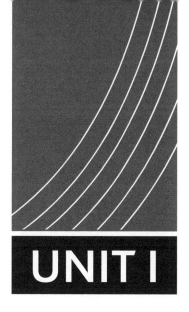

UNIT I

Introduction to Medical Imaging Including Radiographs, CT, Nuclear Scans, MRIs, and Ultrasonography

CHAPTER 1

Radiology Basics

HISTORY OF RADIOLOGY

Understanding not only how radiology began but also how it has progressed through time with the development of various testing modalities in the field of medical imaging will assist the medical provider in their practice. It is most important to gain an understanding of what you are seeing and correlate it with normal physiology as well as pathology. Radiology has been around for more than a century, beginning in November of 1895 when Wilhelm Röentgen discovered the röentgen ray while in his laboratory **(Figure 1.1)**. Dr. Röentgen was a Dutch physicist who published his preliminary findings in a paper titled, "Über eine neue Art von Strahlen (Vorläufige Mittheilung)" or "Over a New Art von Strahlung (Preliminary Communication)" in *Physikalisch-Medizinische Gesellschaft (Physical-Medical Society)* and was awarded the Nobel Prize for physics in 1901. His discovery came during an experiment with cathode ray tubes where it was noted that a fluorescing plate initially shadowed, then portrayed an image of Dr. Röentgen's hand/fingers, and then the hand of his wife with a ring on it **(Figure 1.2)** (Nüsslin, 2020).

The Röentgen ray is invisible and able to penetrate objects, causing it to fluoresce. This ray was originally named by Dr. Röentgen as the *X-Strahlung*, which translates to x-ray.

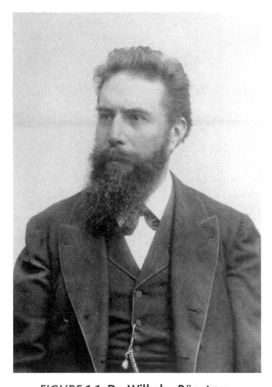

FIGURE 1.1 Dr. Wilhelm Röentgen.

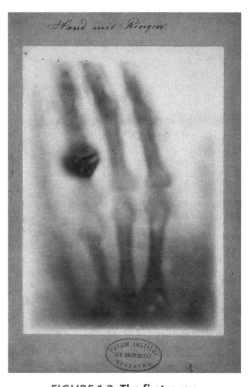

FIGURE 1.2 The first x-ray.

The first clinical x-ray was documented in 1896. Bismuth for stomach x-rays was discovered and utilized to contrast structures not readily seen on a plain radiograph. The dangers of x-rays were first discovered by Dr. Röentgen and his colleagues, and documented in 1901. However, they were not classified as carcinogenic until well after World War II.

Numerous discoveries and "firsts" occurred throughout the 20th century including the modern x-ray tube in 1913, radiographic film in 1918, the automatic processor for film in 1942, and many others. Table 1.1 demonstrates the use of contrast material for stomach x-rays and barium for the gastrointestinal (GI) tract. Other "firsts" during the 20th century

TABLE 1.1 HISTORICAL DISCOVERIES AND FIRSTS IN RADIOLOGY

YEAR	CONTRAST	YEAR	DISCOVERIES	YEAR	FIRSTS
1897	Bismuth for stomach x-rays	1895	Röentgen ray	1896	First clinical x-ray
1910	Barium for GI tract	1913	Modern x-ray tube (hot cathode tube) by William Coolidge	1901	Danger of x-rays
1911	Double contrast for upper GI	1913	Stationary grid by Gustav Bucky	1906	Retrograde pyelogram using silver nitrate
		1913	X-ray film of nitrocellulose	1919	Pneumoencephalogram
				1914-1918	Field hospitals during WWI used radiological equipment
1923	Double contrast for barium enema	1918	Radiographic film	1927	Cerebral angiogram
		1921	Intensifying screens by Carl Patterson	1929	Excretory urogram
		1934	Artificial radionuclides by Frank and Irene Joliot-Curie	1932	Nephrotomography
		1942	Automatic processor for film	1937	Angiocardiogram
		1946	Film cassette changer by George Schoenander	1938	Mammogram
		1946	Nuclear medicine		
		1949	Xerography (dry photocopying also known as electrophotography)	1941	A-mode ultrasound skull

(continued)

TABLE 1.1 HISTORICAL DISCOVERIES AND FIRSTS IN RADIOLOGY *(continued)*

YEAR	CONTRAST	YEAR	DISCOVERIES	YEAR	FIRSTS
		1953	Image intensifier	1948	Coronary artery angiogram
		1957	Whole body nuclear scanner by Hal Anger	1953	Technique for vascular puncture
				1954	Echocardiography
				1962	B-mode ultrasound
				1964	SPECT scanning
				1972	CT scanner
				1974	Positron emission tomography scanner
				1978	Brain MR image
				1980	Commercial MR scanner
				1985	Digital radiography, picture archiving communications and storage system
				1990	Helical CT scanner (spiral)
				1998	Multislice CT scanner
				2000	Molecular imaging
				2000	Digital x-ray detectors used commercially
				2011	3D breast imaging cleared by the FDA
				2014	$12 million grant to the University of Canterbury to build the first human color x-ray scanner in the world

FDA, Food and Drug Administration, GI, gastrointestinal; SPECT, single-photon emission computed tomography; WWII, World War II.

included the first retrograde pyelogram, which was performed in 1906; the first cerebral angiogram in 1927; the first mammogram in 1938; the first A-mode ultrasound in 1941; and the first B-mode ultrasound in 1962. Nuclear medicine was first discovered in 1946, and in 1957 Hal Anger developed a whole-body nuclear scanner. In 1964 the first single-photon emission computed tomography (SPECT) scan was performed. In 1972, the first CT scanner was developed and utilized, with helical scanning capabilities discovered and utilized in 1990. The first commercial MRI scanner was discovered and used to image the brain in 1978. As one can see, medical imaging has come a long way in well over a century and continues to develop and flourish as time progresses.

With the progression from the plain radiograph to the CT scan, MRI, ultrasound, and advancement of nuclear medicine techniques, diagnosing and caring for patients has become more adventitious. Radiographs have assisted providers in identifying changes in air fluid levels, identifying masses, and finding other abnormalities, leading to a more definitive diagnosis. Godfrey Hounsfield invented the principles of CT scanning: With its continued progression into the digital age, this technology has allowed for earlier and more specific findings leading to not only earlier diagnoses but earlier interventions positively affecting outcomes. Ultrasound use began in the 1950s and has rapidly gained acceptance for its real-time images. It has been expanded from not only screening and diagnosis but also assisting in procedures as well as treatments to improve patient outcomes.

Radiology has rapidly advanced since its beginning in 1895. Having an appreciation and understanding of the history of radiological science and its discoveries allows providers to gain an appreciation for diagnostic imaging modalities while ordering and interpreting them daily in practice. An understanding of the testing modalities will also assist providers in choosing, interpreting, and utilizing the findings of the most appropriate test in caring for patients. This, coupled with the American College of Radiology (ACR) Appropriateness Criteria, can assist providers in remaining updated on how best to choose the most cost-effective and appropriate imaging modalities to reduce harm and improve diagnostic specificity.

X-Rays and Image Production

To have an understanding of radiographs and the images that are produced, it is important to learn what an x-ray is. X-Strahlung rays, also known as x-rays, are a form of electromagnetic radiation which, in combination with light, strikes a photosensitive surface; this produces an image that traditionally was processed with chemicals. The radiant energy, which is like visible light or sunlight, is a short wave that is invisible and can penetrate many objects and structures. The shorter the wavelength, the greater its ability to penetrate objects.

Quanta or photons are pockets of energy and are described in terms of particles that travel at the speed of light. Electron volts are a measurement of the amount of energy carried by each photon, which is dependent on the wavelength of the radiation. When an atom loses its electron, it is considered to be ionized. Any photon with 15 or more electron volts is capable of ionization; this is known as ionizing radiation.

X-rays are emitted from a cathode tube. When the rays are released from the tube, they are closely approximated but expand as they travel. The rays then penetrate a structure, striking a cassette on the other side. The amount of radiation that reaches the cassette after penetrating the structure is depicted on a scale from black to white defining the image. The amount of radiation that can penetrate an object is dependent on the amount that is absorbed by the structure, which reduces the amount of energy transmitted through to the cassette (**Figure 1.3**).

Traditionally the cassette held film, which would be processed with chemicals and hung to dry. The images, once they were dry, would then be viewed on a lighted view box or with a hot lamp. If a reading was done prior to the cassette being completely dry it was referred to as a wet reading. There are still areas in the world that continue to use conventional film cassettes. However, with the age of digital technology, the traditional film and cassette has been replaced with digital cassettes, which are processed by an electric reader. This technology has allowed for storing of digital images and sharing of digital images through a picture archiving communications and storage (PACS) system.

Conventional film cassettes consisted of plastic sheets that were coated with an emulsion of silver bromide and iodide that was sensitive to light and radiation. The thin emulsion had a protective coating that, when exposed to ionizing radiation, produced a chemical change.

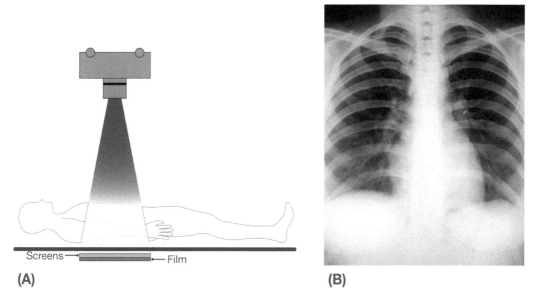

Screens —▭— Film

(A)   (B)

FIGURE 1.3 (A) Release of rays from a cathode tube forming an image. (B) Note that the amount of attenuation causes either black, white, or shades of gray on the image.
Source: (A) Drawing by Ocean City High School student; (B) courtesy of Theresa M. Campo.

The blackness of the film was affected by the amount of radiation reaching it after penetration through an object. If the radiation readily passed through the structure, the area of the film would remain black. The more radiation a structure absorbed, the lighter the structure would appear on the film. The spectrum from black to white on a radiographic image is determined by the amount of radiation absorbed by the density of the specific structure.

Digital cassettes do not use film or chemicals but rather photosensitive electronic plates that have computer-linked detectors; these read measurements of radiation striking various locations, which then form an image. These images are stored and archived and can be shared by numerous providers at various locations, unlike traditional films that were kept in one physical storage location. This has allowed for viewing not only in various locations within a facility or between facilities, but also anywhere digital information can be transmitted. Teleradiology is utilized by some facilities to allow radiologists from opposite sides of the world to read and interpret radiological images and report their findings. This allows for 24-hour accessibility, facilitating expedient results during after-hour and holiday situations.

Radiologic Density

As discussed, during the production of images, the amount of radiation that passes through a structure is captured by the cassette—whether film or digital—thereby producing an image. The scale of black to white is determined by the density of the object, or objects, within the structure. The absorption of the rays by the objects is known as attenuation. Attenuation occurs through a process where the x-rays are removed through absorption or scatter during penetration of the structure (Figure 1.4). If the object is of increased density, then it could absorb the ray as it attempts to pass through.

There are two types of densities that are considered when discussing attenuation and image production in radiology: physical and radiographic. Physical density is the actual thickness and composition of the object or structure that affects the attenuation of the ray as it passes through. Radiographic density is the degree of blackness that is demonstrated

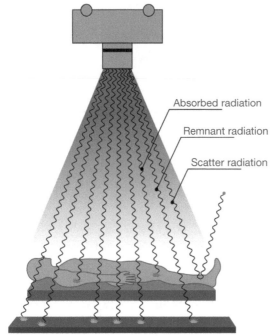

Absorbed radiation

Remnant radiation

Scatter radiation

FIGURE 1.4 **Attenuation of x-rays.**
Source: Drawing by Ocean City High School student.

on the radiographic image and denotes the contrast or differences in density of the radiographic film. Radiographic density of a substance is typically related to its physical density. Physical density can be influenced by the components of the object or structure. For example, the higher the atomic number and metallic component of the object or structure, the more it will cause a white effect in that specific area on the image.

There are four basic densities: air, fat, soft tissue, and bone/metal (Figure 1.5). These four basic densities correspond to the spectrum of black to white on a radiologic image.

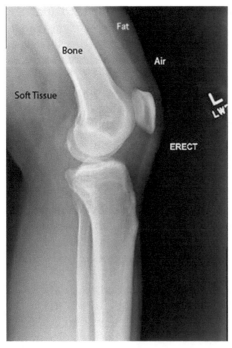

Fat

Bone

Air

Soft Tissue

L

LW

ERECT

FIGURE 1.5 **Four densities on x-ray.**
Source: Courtesy of Dr. David Begleiter; diagramming,
Theresa M. Campo.

Air has a very low density that causes minimal x-ray absorption and produces a black area on the image. Fat produces a dark gray area and soft tissue produces a light gray area on an image. Bone that has a metal component to it from calcium produces a white area on the image. As the density of the object increases, that specific area becomes lighter on the image. The radiologic contrast between soft tissue inclusive of organs, muscles, ligaments, and so forth, is minimal to nonexistent since they are mainly composed of water. The greater the contrast between objects within a structure, the better the visualization of those objects. An example is air within a denser cavity as seen on a chest x-ray of the lungs within the rib cage.

The amount of attenuation corresponds to a unit known as the Hounsfield unit. Air that has little to no absorption has a designation of −1,000 Hounsfield units and is depicted as black on the image. Fat, which has minimal attenuation, is designated as −520 to −100 Hounsfield units and gives a dark gray appearance on the image. Water, which has some attenuation, appears gray on an image, and is designated as 0 Hounsfield units. Soft tissue appears as light gray on an image, since it has more attenuation, and is in the range of 15 to 60 Hounsfield units. Bone, which has a higher attenuation, has a Hounsfield unit at or near 1,000, and appears white on an image (Figure 1.6). Contrast materials such as barium or iodine-based products have a higher Hounsfield unit designation than water; however, they may be comparable or higher than bone. Therefore, they appear to be extremely light or white on the image. Contrast materials are discussed in detail in a later chapter.

Since the discovery of radiology more than a century ago, numerous advancements and innovations have afforded better diagnosis and treatment of disorders. Understanding the science of radiography translates to better interpretation of findings. Knowing the basics of radiology and its shades of gray will help providers distinguish normal from abnormal findings and appreciate what they are visualizing.

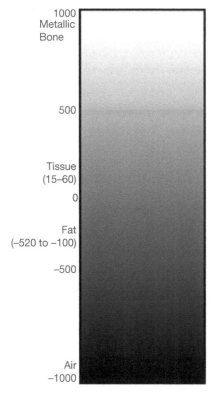

FIGURE 1.6 Hounsfield units.
Source: Drawing by Ocean City High School student.

FACTORS AFFECTING IMAGES

As discussed earlier in this chapter, it is important to understand what produces the spectrum of black to white and the shades of gray in between on a radiologic image. It is also important to appreciate what image effects are intentional or nonintentional. Adequacy of a film is imperative for an accurate reading of any radiological study. Nonintentional factors that can affect a radiological image can occur from physical as well as geometric factors, resulting in thickness, motion, scatter, magnification, and distortion. Intentional factors include those that are planned to highlight an area for evaluation with contrast enhancement.

Nonintentional Factors

The thickness of an object and its physical density can affect the attenuation of the rays attempting to penetrate that object or structure. The thicker the object, the more radiation is needed to penetrate that specific object. Conversely, the smaller or thinner an object, the less radiation is needed to penetrate that specific object (Figure 1.7). It is imperative that the appropriate dose of radiation be used to penetrate the object based on its thickness. If the same amount of radiation is utilized with a study on an 80-pound patient as opposed to a 500-pound patient, the image may be over- or underpenetrated. When an image is under- or overpenetrated, there will be inadequate contrast, resulting in a suboptimal image as key structures may fail to be differentiated and visualized.

Another factor resulting in distortion is motion. Motion can result in a blurry or hazy image that may not be able to be interpreted. As an object moves, the penetrating rays become absorbed by the structure at different rates, making the image appear hazy or blurred (Figure 1.8). Motion artifact can be corrected with shortened exposure times.

Scatter is a deflection of the primary radiation beam and produces a foggy image (Figure 1.9). There are processes that can be used to reduce scatter and eliminate shadows that may occur. The Bucky–Potter system is a method that uses a grid with alternating angled slats that are very thin and radiolucent combined with thin lead strips. Rapid movement of the whole grid during exposure helps eliminate shadows and scatter.

Magnification may be altered if an object is not the appropriate distance from the cassette. The farther away an object is from the film or detector plate, the greater the magnification of that object. This can reduce the sharpness of contrast, making it difficult to interpret the

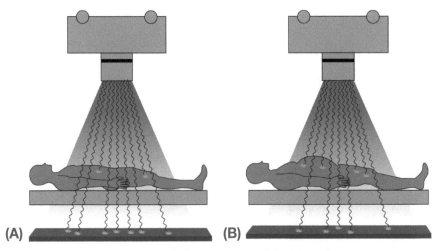

FIGURE 1.7 (A) Small versus (B) large person.
Source: Drawing by Ocean City High School student.

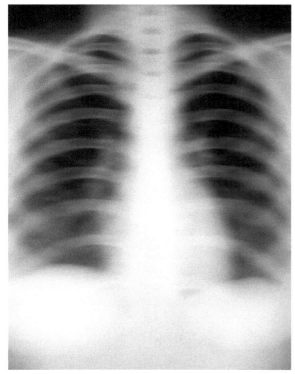

FIGURE 1.8 Effect of motion causing a blurry image.
Source: Courtesy of Dr. Keith Lafferty.

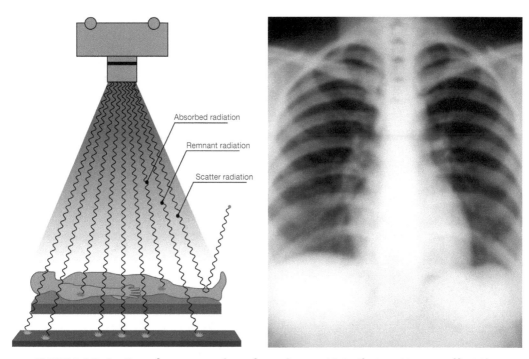

Absorbed radiation

Remnant radiation

Scatter radiation

FIGURE 1.9 Scatter of x-rays causing a foggy image. Note that scatter can affect the appearance of the image.
Source: (Left) Drawing by Ocean City High School student; (right) courtesy of Dr. Keith Lafferty.

images (**Figure 1.10**). Magnification can also be altered by the direction where the ray enters and exits the structure. For example, in a posterior to anterior view, the beam of radiation penetrates the structure from back to front. If the direction is changed from to anterior to posterior, even if the beam is going in the same direction, magnification of the beam as it reaches the other end of the structure will be altered (**Figure 1.11**).

It is also important that the beam be perpendicular to the film or detector plate. When a beam is not perpendicular, distortion of the image occurs, affecting the clarity and appearance of structures.

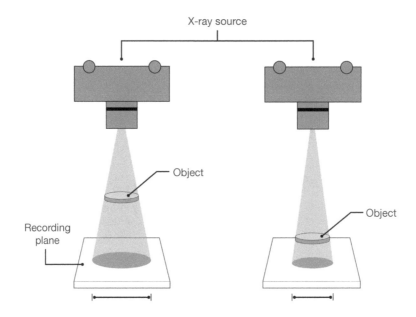

FIGURE 1.10 The effect of magnification on an image. Note that the farther away an object is from the cassette, the larger it becomes. The same is true as the beam travels through the body.
Source: Drawing by Ocean City High School student.

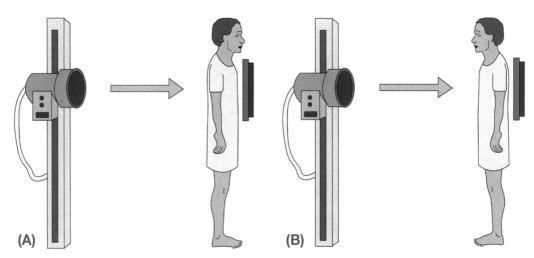

FIGURE 1.11 (A) Posterior–anterior versus (B)anterior–posterior view.
Source: Drawing by Ocean City High School student.

Intentional Effects

Intentional effects of an image can be obtained with the use of contrast material. Contrast material allows for increased contrast of a particular object within a structure for easier visualization (Figure 1.12). Contrast may be used to examine structures that typically would not be seen on a normal radiograph. Contrast was used more extensively in the past in conjunction with standard x-rays before the invention of CT and MRI to evaluate abdominal, pelvic, or intracranial abnormalities. Contrast consists of elements such as barium and iodine-based products that allow for better visualization of structures in radiographs and CT imaging or paramagnetic agents used in MRI studies.

There are two types of contrast used for radiographs: barium and iodinated benzene ring solutions, such as gastrografin. Barium is used to visualize areas of the GI tract, specifically to better visualize the mucosa in detail. It is also beneficial in visualizing the luminal wall of the bowel. It can be given by mouth for an antegrade study or rectally for a retrograde study. Barium sulfate has a high atomic weight, which increases its radiological density; this causes a white effect on the film. Oral contrast is generally not absorbed and, therefore, does not pose a risk of allergic reaction. It is resistant to dilution, which is why it is not recommended for the evaluation of large bowel obstruction or perforation. If the contrast remains in the bowel for a prolonged period, it becomes thickened and can cause the obstruction to become worse. It is contraindicated in perforation because it reacts with and incites granulomatous changes in the peritoneum. It can also interfere with subsequent studies such as CT scans, making them nondiagnostic. If a perforation is present, then the contrast can leak out of the bowel, potentially causing a desmoplastic reaction.

Water-soluble contrast containing iodide should be used if perforation or large bowel obstruction is suspected. Water-soluble contrast does not cause a desmoplastic reaction if leaked into surrounding areas and is absorbed and excreted by the kidney. The basic

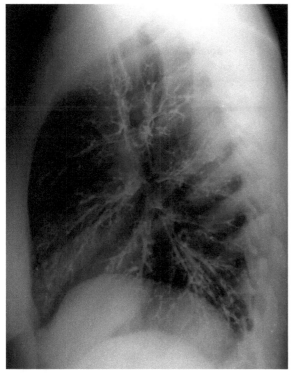

FIGURE 1.12 **Contrasted study. Note the ability to visualize the small airways otherwise not seen with a plain radiograph.**
Source: Radiopaediageneral@radiopaedia.org

structure of water-soluble contrast is an iodinated benzene ring that also has a high atomic number, causing increased contrast and differentiation of structures not readily visualized on the plain radiograph.

Water-soluble contrast can be injected to highlight organs, vessels, and abnormalities. Angiography, myelography, arthropathy, and urography studies also use water-soluble contrast for indirect contrast imaging. Water-soluble contrast is contraindicated if an esophageal airway fistula is suspected or if one is at risk of aspiration, since leakage into lung tissue can cause a severe and devastating chemical pneumonia. If extravasation of the material occurs during IV infusion, tissue necrosis can result. Treatment for this adverse effect includes removing the IV catheter immediately, elevating the site, and applying warm or cold compresses to reduce swelling. If a large volume of contrast extravasates into the tissue, surgical intervention may be required.

There are many uses of contrast to enhance a radiographic image. Urographic studies to visualize the genitourinary (GU) tract involve administering water-soluble contrast either intravenously or through the urethra and into the bladder and renal pelvis, utilizing a retrograde method. The use of IV urography is replacing the use of CT scanning.

Angiography is used to image circulatory flow within an organ or structure. For these studies, water-soluble media is injected either intravenously or intra-arterially and then a series of images is performed demonstrating circulatory flow within the structure. A sonogram or fistulogram is performed to identify abnormal sinus tracts in the body by injecting contrast material within the suspected area. Inserting a needle between the spinal processes of the lumbar vertebrae entering the subarachnoid space and injecting a water-soluble contrast material under fluoroscopic monitoring is a myelogram.

One of the risks with water-soluble contrast agents is allergic reaction. Any persons allergic to iodine-based products should either be premedicated prior to the start of the study or an alternative radiologic evaluation should be considered to avoid a negative outcome. Allergy to shellfish is considered a risk for reaction to water-soluble contrast agents. However, limited evidence shows an actual correlation. Patients with poor renal function or severe dehydration may be at increased risk for contrast-induced nephropathy. Therefore, these patients should not be exposed to water-soluble contrast material. Patients who are dehydrated, have diabetes, and those having borderline renal function should receive IV hydration before and after receiving water-soluble contrast, if an alternative modality is not available. Additionally, patients taking metformin with known borderline kidney function are also at increased risk for life-threatening lactic acidosis when receiving water-soluble contrast since metformin is normally cleared by renal tubular secretion.

Paramagnetic agents are used as contrast material with MRI, which helps to better define abnormalities and differentiate disease processes (i.e., herniated nuclear pulposis [HNP] from scars). There are two types of paramagnetic agents—gadolinium (Gd) and gadolinium-diethylenetriaminepentaacetic acid (Gd-DTPA). Free gadolinium is not used. Gadolinium gives greater detail to soft tissue and vascular structures. However, Gd-DTPA is the most used paramagnetic agent due to its strong effect on the relaxation time during the scanning sequence. Relaxation time will be discussed in Chapter 3. Gadolinium can be mixed with iodinated contrasting agents useful in needle localization.

Adverse and allergic reactions rarely occur with paramagnetic contrast agents, and the risk of anaphylaxis and allergic reaction with the use of these agents is lower than those caused by iodinated contrasting agents. Nephrogenic systemic fibrosis is a rarely occurring adverse reaction that can occur with paramagnetic contrast agents. Nephrogenic systemic fibrosis causes a progressive tissue change in skin, joints, eyes, and internal organs that occurs more frequently in patients with renal insufficiency and failure.

CONCLUSION

Contrast agents can be very beneficial in differentiating structures with similar density that normally would not be visualized on an imaging study. They are also useful in identifying abnormalities such as masses, tumors, fistulas, and HNP, resulting in a more timely therapeutic intervention. Further discussion of the use of contrast agents with various studies is presented in the chapters on the five testing modalities of plain radiographs, CT, MRI, ultrasound, and nuclear imaging.

RESOURCES

American College of Radiology. (n.d.). *Appropriateness criteria.* http://www.acr.org/quality-safety/appropriateness-criteria

Au-Yong, I., Au-Yong, A., & Broderick, N. (2010). *On-call x-rays made easy.* Churchill Livingstone, Elsevier.

Brant, W. E. (2012). Diagnostic imaging methods. In W. E. Brant & C. A. Helms (Eds.), *Fundamentals of diagnostic radiology* (4th ed., pp. 2–27). Wolters Kluwer/Lippincott Williams & Wilkins.

Daffner, R. H. (2014). Overview and principles of diagnostic imaging. In R. H. Daffner & M. S. Hartman (Eds.), *Clinical radiology: The essentials* (4th ed., pp. 1–42). Wolters Kluwer/Lippincott Williams & Wilkins.

Daffner, R. H., & Hartman, R. H. (2014). Radiographic contrast agents. In R. H. Daffner & M. S. Hartman (Eds.), *Clinical radiology: The essentials* (4th ed., pp. 43–48). Wolters Kluwer/Lippincott Williams & Wilkins.

Herring, W. (2016). *Learning radiology: Recognizing the basics* (3rd ed., pp. 1–7). Elsevier.

Nett, B. (n.d.). *History x-ray imaging: radiography, fluoroscopy, mammography. How radiology works.* https://howradiologyworks.com/history-xray-imaging/

No Author. (2021). *History of radiology: Timeline, pioneers, inventions.* https://www.ramsoft.com/history-of-radiology/

Nüsslin, F. (2020). Wilhelm Conrad Röentgen: The scientist and his discovery. *Review Paper,* 79, 65–68. https://doi.org/10.1016/j.ejmp.2020.10.010. https://www.physicamedica.com/article/S1120-1797(20)30253-2/fulltext

Taylor, C. R. (2015). *Abdominal computed tomography scanning.* http://emedicine.medscape.com/article/2114236-overview

CHAPTER 2

Radiating Testing Modalities

This chapter introduces and briefly discusses the different radiological testing modalities that use ionizing radiation. The section on each testing modality describes how the images are obtained by the various machines and technology, their uses and benefits, as well as the downfalls associated with each modality. This allows for differentiating the various modalities, but also gives an appreciation for how the images are produced. Knowledge of the various testing modalities is fundamental in understanding the most cost-effective and appropriate diagnostic studies for suspected conditions.

RADIOGRAPHS

Radiographs have been used for more than a century, revolutionizing current medical imaging. Since their invention in 1895, radiographs have been used to identify and diagnose abnormalities so that treatments can be provided. The increased use of radiographs has improved lives through early detection of conditions leading to further studies and/or treatments of identified diseases. Radiology science has led to the development of more precise testing modalities such as computed tomography (CT), magnetic resonance imaging (MRI), nuclear medicine, and ultrasonography.

Radiographs can be either plain, meaning there is no contrast enhancement, or they can be a contrast study (Figure 2.1). Plain radiographs are ideal for identifying gross abnormalities and foreign bodies, visualizing calculi and fractures, or evaluating air, fluid, and gas patterns. They are advantageous because they are inexpensive, nonoperator dependent, and readily available as they can be obtained via a designated radiology room, a portable machine, or a mobile unit such as a mobile mammography bus. One of the disadvantages of radiography is its limited ability to contrast densities of organs and tissue.

Radiographs are performed utilizing a single view. This means that the x-rays are emitted from the cathode tube and directed toward a cassette on the other side of the patient. The direction of the beam penetrating the patient is how that view is labeled. When we have a posterior–anterior (PA) view, the tube is behind (or posterior, hence "P") the patient who is standing or sitting erect with the cassette directly in front of them. The x-ray beam then travels from the tube, penetrating from the back to the front (or anterior, hence "A") of the patient. The image is then produced on the cassette in front of the patient (Figure 2.2A). In the anterior–posterior (AP) view, the opposite occurs (Figure 2.2B). This distinction is important: Recall from Chapter 1 the magnification of objects caused by their distance from the plate. The image is also labeled based on the position of the patient, such as erect, supine, prone, or decubitus. In the lateral decubitus view, the patient lies on their side for at least 3 to 5 minutes to allow any free air to rise and is then imaged in a side-lying position (Figure 2.2C).

In 2015, the first colored images were published demonstrating the ability of a computer to detect the different wavelengths of x-rays that pass through different structures (Figure 2.3)

Contrast can be used to highlight areas of interest such as the intestines, bladder, kidneys, vessels, and so on. Contrasted studies can be static or dynamic. Static images are

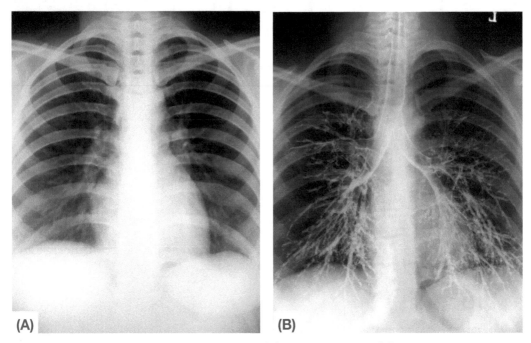

(A)   (B)

FIGURE 2.1 Plain versus contrasted study: (A) plain radiograph; (B) contrast radiograph. Notice how the contrast highlights the airways that are normally not visualized on plain film.
Source: Courtesy of Dr. Frank Gaillard, Radiopaedia.org.

stationary images in a one plane view. Dynamic images give real-time radiographic visualization of moving anatomical structures such as the heart and diaphragm. These are performed using fluoroscopy, which can be either diagnostic or therapeutic. Therapeutic uses can include cardiac catheterization with stent placements, injections into the spinal canal, or vascular line placements.

Fluoroscopy involves a fluoroscopic screen combined with an electronic device that converts visible light into an electron score stream. This technique amplifies the image, making it brighter, and then converts it back into visible light. When fluoroscopy is performed, the x-ray tube lies beneath the table. With the tube beneath the table, the cassette is then supported over the top of the table and the patient is positioned for the study or therapeutic intervention (Figure 2.4). The study may be labeled based on the patient's position relative to the tube. For example, a right posterior oblique indicates the patient was lying with the right side down, back against the table, at an angle greater than 0° and less than 90° with the tube beneath and the cassette overhead.

Radiographs have revolutionized medicine since their discovery in 1895, leading to new testing modalities such as the CT scan, nuclear scan, MRI, and ultrasonography. With the utilization of plain and contrast radiographs, patients are being diagnosed earlier with abnormalities and disorders that can now be treated earlier and more definitively. Technological advances will surely lead to more enhanced testing modalities and better and safer testing modalities in the future.

There are many benefits to radiographs such as cost, ease of ordering, and ease of interpretation, as well as utilization of contrast studies. However, the clarity and definition gained through other radiologic testing such as CT and MRI have led to a decreased use of contrast radiographs, for example, barium enema. Radiographs are limited by single views and limited contrasting of structures that are overcome with the use of cross-sectional imaging of the body with CT, MRI, and ultrasonography, which will be discussed in this chapter and in Chapter 3.

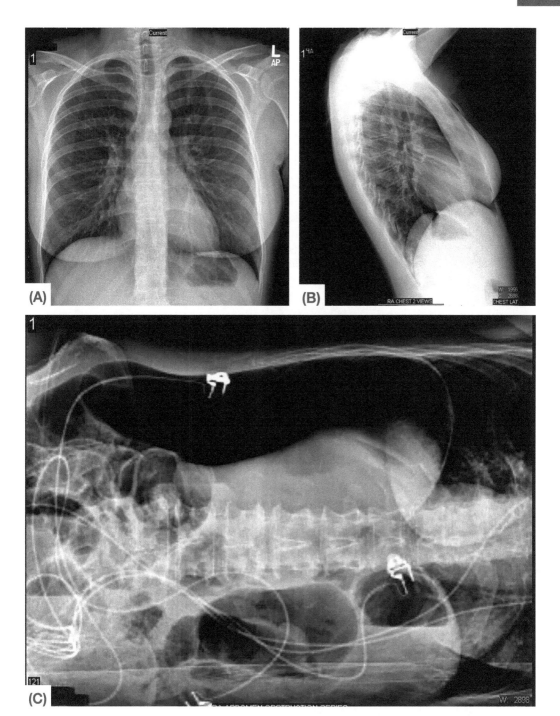

FIGURE 2.2 (A) Normal chest posterior–anterior view; (B) normal chest lateral view; and (C) decubitus view. Note the air/fluid levels on the decubitus view.
Source: (A) and (B) courtesy of Theresa M. Campo; (C) courtesy of Dr. Keith Lafferty.

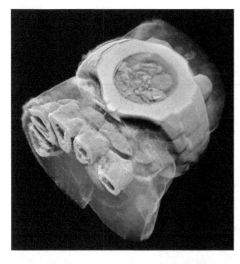

FIGURE 2.3 A human wrist (and wristwatch) imaged with the new 3D, color x-ray machine developed by MARS Bioimaging.
Source: Mars Bioimaging, http://www.marsbioimaging.com.

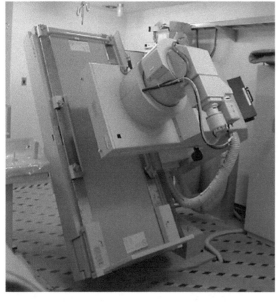

FIGURE 2.4 Fluoroscopic procedure table.
Source: https://commons.wikimedia.org/wiki/File:Fluoroscope.jpg

COMPUTED TOMOGRAPHY

CT, also known as computed axial tomography (CAT) scanning, was first introduced by Sir Godfrey Hounsfield and Dr. Allan Cormack around 1974. The word *tomography* is derived from the Greek word "tomos," meaning "section." Radiographs produce only one image of one two-dimensional plane from one beam. However, CT scans can produce multiple slices, allowing for reproducible images in 3D planes.

CT scanners employ an x-ray beam that rotates along a circular pattern with detectors rotating along the opposite side. This allows for the system to move in a 360° circle with a well collimated or restricted beam. The beam only travels in one direction through the patient to the detector on the opposite side (Figure 2.5). A complex computer system utilizes algorithms and mathematical formulas to process the data into a large number of 2D slices, like images that can then be formatted into multiple reconstructed planes. The data analyzed by the computer system then assign Hounsfield units (HU) to reconstruct the image based on geometrical plots.

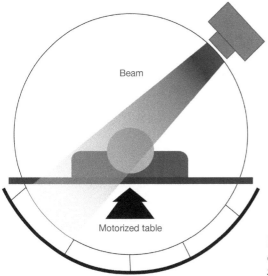

Beam

Motorized table

FIGURE 2.5 CT scanner showing 360° of circle detectors and beams.
Source: Drawing by Ocean City High School student.

Images are composed of a matrix of thousands of tiny squares called pixels. The pixels have a computer-assigned number that correlates to an HU. As discussed earlier, this scale is what produces the shades of gray from black to white. HUs are not absolute and may vary from one CT system to another,ranging from −1,000 to +1,000 HU. However, they can also range from −1,024 to +3,000 or 4,000 HU.

During a CT scan, the patient is placed on a table and the x-ray beam and detector system move through 360° around them. The detectors receive the x-rays and measure the amount of absorption of the rays as they pass through the body. These data are obtained by the computer and then analyzed and assigned a HU. The computer then produces an image based on the geometric plots of pixels (which are based on the absorption and scatter of the x-ray), resulting in an image on the screen. When viewing the results, the appearance of the images is dependent on the window and level used to display the image. The window describes the range of HUs displayed, and the level describes the center of the window. The wider (or larger) the window, the more types of densities will be displayed; however, the difference between similar types of tissue lessens, making tissue differentiation difficult to discriminate. The level and window are displayed on every CT image.

The CT image is made up of multiple individual boxes, called pixels. The CT pixel number is proportional to the differences in attenuation of the x-ray by the tissue and is compared with water. The number of pixels can be changed, but they are typically in a matrix (such as 256 × 256). Each image will also have a slice thickness, and the 2D slice will represent all the densities within the volume. The volume of tissue represented by the pixel is called a voxel. The forecastle allows for reconstruction of images by the computer system without losing resolution of the image. Voxel dimensions are determined by the computer system utilizing algorithms that are chosen for the type of reconstruction and are based on the thickness of the scanned slices. If a particular tissue, organ, or lesion is of increased density, then there will be increased absorption, resulting in increased attenuation of the x-ray beam. The more a substance attenuates the beam, the more radiopaque or radiodense it is said to be. On the black and white scale of images on a CT, typically the more radiodense an object is, the closer to white it is displayed. If the particular objects are of decreased density, then there will be decreased absorption of the ray or decreased attenuation, causing a black appearance on the image that is known as radiolucency. You may hear of objects described this way, with a radiodense object being called either a "high density" object (such as a stone or calcification) or a "low density" object (such as gas or fat).

The axial view is the traditional view obtained by the CT scanner. With the ability to reconstruct images, the computer system can include sagittal, coronal, and oblique planes (Figure 2.6). CT computer systems also utilize volumetric data to produce a 3D image during the reconstruction process (Figure 2.7). This is due to the ability to produce volumetric data sets. 3D reconstruction is because of the higher speed scanning of multislice CT and increased computer processing speed and ability.

Conventional single-slice scanners were much slower than the technology utilized today with helical or spiral scanners. This is because the patient would hold their breath while a single slice was taken and then release their breath. The table would then move and this would be repeated. This produced images in slices or sections.

Currently, helical or spiral scanners are utilized to acquire images. These systems allow the table to move at a constant speed, which allows for a more rapid study. Modern systems also include multidetectors, allowing for data to be acquired using rows of detectors that rotate at one time. Multidetector and multislice systems and technology allow for additional studies to be derived from the data obtained in one study. An advantage of current CT scanners is their ability for rapid scan acquisition. This rapid scanning allows for larger areas to be scanned in less time with greater resolution. That means that breathing

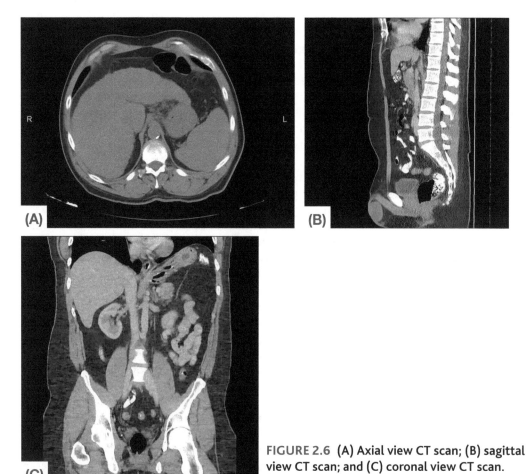

FIGURE 2.6 (A) Axial view CT scan; (B) sagittal view CT scan; and (C) coronal view CT scan.
Source: Courtesy of Dr. David Begleiter.

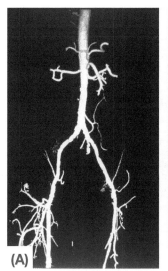
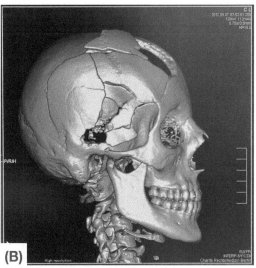

FIGURE 2.7 (A) and (B) 3D CT image.
Source: (A) Courtesy of Dr. David Begleiter. (B)
Courtesy of Prof. Dr. Michael Tsokos, https://commons.wikimedia.org/wiki/File:12-06-11-rechtsmedizin-berlin-07.jpg.

and motion artifacts are greatly reduced; there is greater resolution of images, allowing smaller and smaller objects to be visualized and even allowing scanning of certain areas, such as the coronary arteries, which were never before possible. They also allow for accurate multiplane and 3D reconstruction (this is true of any CT, whether single or multislice).

CT fluoroscopy can be used with current CT scanners (another advantage of multislice CT). Fluoroscopy improves the performance of image-guided procedures such as biopsies, drainage, and other interventional procedures and is of particular use in guiding needle placement in the chest and abdomen, areas that are prone to movement. These CT scans may also be enhanced with the use of contrast, either IV, oral, or rectal. Oral and rectal routes are beneficial in visualizing and identifying the bowel and its abnormalities. IV contrast is helpful in enhancing vascular anatomy, demonstrating vessel patency and integrity, and identification of lesions or masses and improves the ability to characterize them. IV contrast can also improve the visualization of solid organs such as the liver and spleen. Enhancement assists in differentiating normal anatomy from pathology.

As with radiographs, CT images can be affected by many factors. Artifact has the greatest impact on the clarity of an image. There are many types of artifacts that can affect image quality. If a patient voluntarily or involuntarily moves during the study, it can affect the image, causing prominent streaks from higher to lower density that appear as blurring or shadowing of structures. Metal objects such as surgical clips, staples, and dental fillings can cause streak artifacts because the computer systems are not able to distinguish between high-density sharp-edged objects and adjoining lower density structures. Beam hardening artifacts may be seen as areas of streaking on images, whereas ring artifacts can demonstrate high- or low-density circular rings on the image **(Figure 2.8)**.

CT scans are extremely beneficial in diagnosing critical abnormalities and producing real-time images. This allows for CT-guided procedures and fluoroscopy because of the rapid obtaining of images with multislice and multidetector scanners. With the advancements in technology, computer systems allow providers to view areas of interest in multiple plains, including 3D images.

In 2021, the Food and Drug Administration (USFDA, 2021) cleared the first imaging device for CT. The technology utilizes photo-counting detectors in place of the current

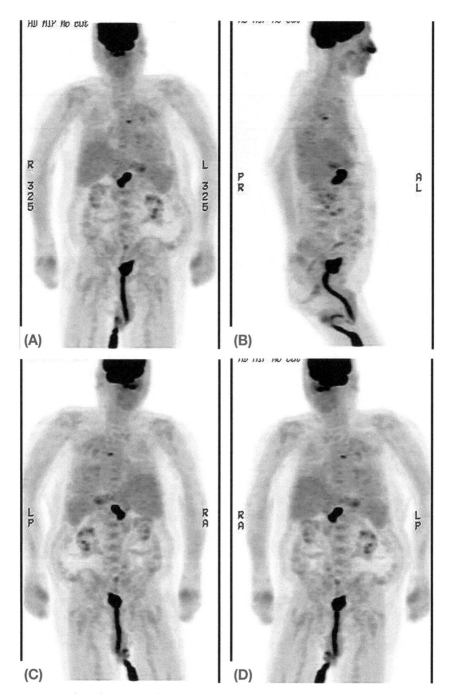

FIGURE 2.8 (A–D) Positive (positive electron) emission tomography scan images.
Source: Courtesy of Dr. David Begleiter.

detectors measuring each individual x-ray passing through the body instead of measuring the total energy contained in x-rays producing a more detailed image. Most recently a university in Munich has integrated dark-field x-rays with CT scanners to produce 3D x-ray images. Dark-field x-rays emit very low radiation doses and produce finer detailed images by visualizing scattering of x-rays in tissues (Pfeiffer, n.d.). Technology for producing low-dose high-quality CT scan images is a current priority whether for screening or diagnosing.

NUCLEAR SCANNING

Nuclear medicine scans and their images are both diagnostic and therapeutic. Nuclear imaging for diagnostic purposes involves a radioactive isotope, an unstable form of an element that emits radiation from its nucleus as it decays, resulting in a stable, but nonradioactive product. Radioactive isotopes occur naturally and artificially. Uranium and thorium are examples of naturally occurring radioactive isotopes. Artificial radioactive isotopes can occur through either neutron enrichment in a nuclear reactor or within a cyclotron. Radioactive isotopes are low dose, nontoxic, and have a short half-life. They are readily incorporated into physiologic compounds and are relatively inexpensive. Technetium-99m is the most widely used radioisotope in imaging studies.

Radioisotopes are combined and attached to inert agents with binding properties, allowing for concentration in body tissues. Various tissues and organs absorb substances differently. For example, the thyroid best absorbs iodine, the brain best absorbs glucose, and bones best absorb phosphate. Radiopharmaceuticals are referred to as radionuclides, radio tracers, or simply tracers. Most are carried to tissues or organs by the bloodstream; then gamma camera imaging is used to measure radioactive emission. Some agents may be given orally or inhaled, as in ventilation/perfusion (V/Q) scans, or instilled in the bladder for reflux studies. In its simplest form, the gamma camera records radiation emissions from a patient in a single view or plane at point; in its more advanced form, the gamma camera rotates around the patient, acquiring several 2D images from multiple angles. The 2D images are then reconstructed into a 3D data set by a computer. This is known as single-photon emission computed tomography (SPECT).

Positron (positive electron) emission tomography (PET) produces a 3D image depicting the body's biochemistry and metabolic processes at a molecular level. The positive electron or positron radioisotope is attached to a pharmaceutical used in the body's metabolism. This radiopharmaceutical is taken up proportionally with how metabolically active the tissue is. This technique is useful in diagnosing cancer; it is also useful following changes resulting from therapeutic interventions, creating the ability to identify hidden metastasis and recurrence. The PET cyclotron, or generator, produces isotopes with a relatively short half-life that emit positrons. Positrons are significantly higher energy particles that are recorded and used to produce PET images. In general, positron emission generates far less radiation exposure than CT scans or fluoroscopy. However, cardiac PET scanning is known to generate the greatest amount of radiation exposure among all nuclear studies. **Figure 2.9** shows examples of PET scan images.

As stated earlier, the half-life is generally shorter with radioisotopes than with other agents. Generally, there are three ways to describe the half-life of a radioisotope. The physical half-life is the period in which an element would decay naturally on its own whether it is sitting on the shelf in a container or if it has been administered; that is, the time at which half of the original radioactivity is gone. The biologic half-life is based on the normal physiologic removal of the radioisotope and the pharmaceutical. For example, when it is excreted from the kidneys and/or the GI tract, the biologic half-life is shorter than the natural physical half-life. Finally, effective half-life is a mathematical derivation based on formulas that combine biologic and physical parameters. It is a measurement of when the actual isotope remains effective within the body.

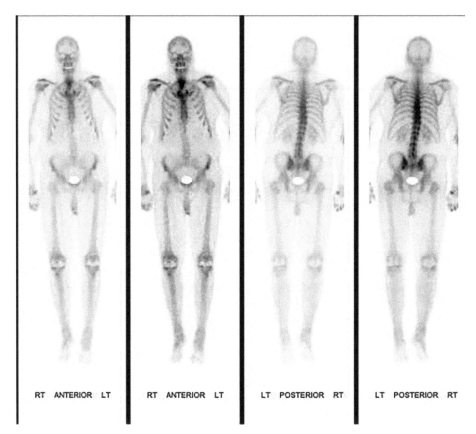

FIGURE 2.9 Static image bone scans.
Source: Courtesy of Dr. David Begleiter.

PET scanning can be used in conjunction with a CT scan to give a more accurate localization of an abnormality or lesion for surgery or biopsy, or to identify suspected metastasis. When PET and SPECT CT scanning are performed together, there is an increased specificity and sensitivity in the cardiac, neural, and oncological identification of abnormalities. These enhanced imaging modalities also improve the identification of malignancies and staging of treatment in cancer patients.

Nuclear imaging is unique in its ability to provide high functional resolution, providing physiologic as well as functional information of organ structure that is not otherwise available with CT, MRI, or ultrasound imaging. Functional imaging identifies whether an organ is functioning normally or abnormally, independent from anatomical abnormalities.

Two types of images can be obtained with a nuclear study: static or dynamic. Static images evaluate organs and areas in a still state, such as thyroid scans, liver scans, splenic scans, and so on **(Figure 2.10)**. Dynamic images include rapid sequence images of moving areas such as blood flow to organs, muscles of the skeleton, and renal perfusion. Nuclear imaging is based on the detection and mapping of the biodistribution of radio tracers that have been administered and captured by emission imaging. Table 2.1 demonstrates the five basic isotope concentrations in the body, the mechanism, the type of study, what is assessed in that study, and what is absorbed by that organ with consideration of radioisotopes attaching to pharmaceuticals.

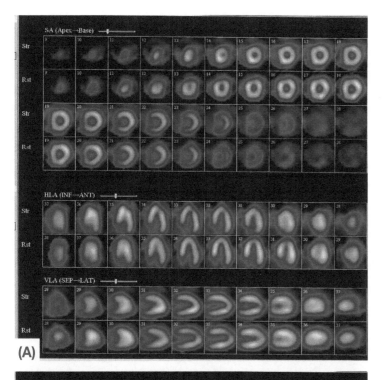

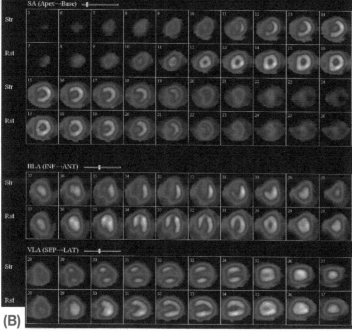

FIGURE 2.10 (A) Dynamic image; pre-exercise nuclear stress test; (B) large antero apical and septal ischemia. Note loss of areas in all three views compared to a normal scan.
Source: Courtesy of Dr. Yatish B. Merchant.

Nuclear imaging allows for identification of abnormal tissue, such as cancer and metastasis, and provides imaging, reflecting the functionality of an organ and/or system. Innovations in the field of nuclear imaging include molecular medicine and molecular imaging, applying genomics and protein messaging that allow the following of gene

TABLE 2.1 THE FIVE BASIC ISOTOPE CONCENTRATIONS IN THE BODY

TYPE OF ISOTOPE CONCENTRATION	SCAN	ABSORPTION	EVALUATES
Blood pool or compartment localization	Cardiac	Glucose	Perfusion
			Function
			Viability
	Brain		Mass
Physiological inclusion	Thyroid	Iodine	Goiter
			Hyperthyroid
			Cancer
	Bone	Phosphates	Metastasis
			Abuse
Capillary blockage	Lung		Pulmonary embolus (obstruction)
			Quantitative perfusion
Phagocytosis	Liver		Cholestasis
			Mass
			Metastasis
Cell sequestration	Spleen		Injury
			Mass

therapy as well as stem cell therapy from its introduction into the patient. The capabilities of nuclear imaging allow the diagnosis of abnormalities and can measure therapeutic effects so interventions can be modified based on the patient's response. As with CT scans, advances in nuclear scanning technology focus on reducing radiation dose and increasing resolution and image quality.

CONCLUSION

The three radiating testing modalities are similar in how the image is obtained. However, CT and nuclear imaging take this foundation further with multiple views, contrast, and digital technology. When deciding on the appropriate testing modality to order, it is important to take into consideration how the images are obtained and what you are looking to achieve.

Consideration must be given to the amount of radiation exposure a patient receives from every radiological study. The risk and benefit as well as the necessity of each study must be weighed carefully to protect patients. A radiation dose of 50 millisieverts (mSv) can place a person at risk for cancer. A CT of the abdomen and pelvis can emit approximately 30 mSv when performed with and without contrast. Correlation of cancer to radiation exposure can take one to two decades, making it difficult to determine the actual risk.

RESOURCES

American College of Radiology. (n.d.). *Appropriateness criteria*. Retrieved July 11, 2023, from http://www.acr.org/quality-safety/appropriateness-criteria

Au-Yong, I., Au-Yong, A., & Broderick, N. (2010). *On-call x-rays made easy*. Churchill Livingstone, Elsevier.

Badawi, R. D., Kroger, L. A., & Bushberg, J. T. (2012). Essential science of nuclear medicine. In W. E. Brant & C. A. Helms (Eds.), *Fundamentals of diagnostic radiology* (4th ed., pp. 1233–1249). Wolters Kluwer/Lippincott Williams & Wilkins.

Brant, W. E. (2012). Diagnostic imaging methods. In W. E. Brant & C. A. Helms (Eds.), *Fundamentals of diagnostic radiology* (4th ed., pp. 2–27). Wolters Kluwer/Lippincott Williams & Wilkins.

Cameron, C. F., Bijan, B., & Shelton, D. K. (2012). Positron emission tomography. In W. E. Brant & C. A. Helms (Eds.), *Fundamentals of diagnostic radiology* (4th ed., pp. 1388–1419). Wolters Kluwer/Lippincott Williams & Wilkins.

Daffner, R. H. (2014). Overview and principles of diagnostic imaging. In R. H. Daffner & M. S. Hartman (Eds.), *Clinical radiology: The essentials* (4th ed., pp. 1–42). Wolters Kluwer/Lippincott Williams & Wilkins.

Daffner, R. H., & Hartman, R. H. (2014). Radiographic contrast agents. In R. H. Daffner & M. S. Hartman (Eds.), *Clinical radiology: The essentials* (4th ed., pp. 43–48). Wolters Kluwer/Lippincott Williams & Wilkins.

Donnelly, L. F. (2009). *Pediatric imaging: The fundamentals*. Saunders Elsevier.

Herring, W. (2016). *Learning radiology: Recognizing the basics* (3rd ed., pp. 1–7). Elsevier.

Pfeiffer, F. (n.d.). *Grating based x-ray dark field imaging: Method causes scattering of x-rays in tissue*. Munich Institute of Biomedical Engineering Technical University of Munich. https://www.bioengineering.tum.de/en/research/microscopy-and-biomedical-imaging/grating-based-x-ray-dark-field-imaging

Pfeiffer, F. (2022). *New technology for clinical CT scans: Prototype of a clinical CT device combines dark-field x-ray and conventional technology*. Technical University of Munich. https://www.eurekalert.org/news-releases/942783

Shelton, D. K. (2012). Introduction to nuclear medicine. In W. E. Brant & C. A. Helms (Eds.), *Fundamentals of diagnostic radiology* (4th ed., pp. 1228–1232). Wolters Kluwer/Lippincott Williams & Wilkins.

U.S. Food and Drug Administration. (2021). *FDA clears first major imaging device advancement for computed tomography in nearly a decade*. https://www.fda.gov/news-events/press-announcements/fda-clears-first-major-imaging-device-advancement-computed-tomography-nearly-decade#:~:text=The%20device%20uses%20the%20emerging,many%20X%2Drays%20at%20once

CHAPTER 3

Nonradiating Testing Modalities

This chapter introduces and briefly discusses the two testing modalities that do not use ionizing radiation to produce an image. Each testing modality is described, including how the images are obtained by the various machines and technology, their uses and benefits, and their limitations. This allows for differentiating the various modalities and provides an appreciation for how the images are produced. Understanding the various testing modalities is fundamental in deciding what tests are most useful for diagnostic purposes.

MAGNETIC RESONANCE IMAGING

Magnetic resonance imaging (MRI) was simultaneously discovered by two physicists, Felix Bloch and Edward Mills Purcell, in the late 1940s; both men won the Nobel Prize in 1952 for their discovery. However, it was not until the late 1970s when Paul Lauterbur, Peter Mansfield, and Raymond Damadian began using MRIs and clinical images in the diagnostic study of patients.

The science behind MRI is quite different from that of radiographs and CT scans. MRI does not use ionizing radiation for the development of images but rather uses the inherent magnetism of tissues, especially hydrogen in water, which constitutes approximately 70% of the human body. MRI scanners use very strong magnetic fields and radiofrequency waves to manipulate the electromagnetic activity of protons within the hydrogen nucleus. The radiofrequency waves influence the spin of the protons used to produce the image, changing the magnetic fields. The energy released in this process is then received by coils in the scanner and processed by a computer to form an image (Figure 3.1).

An MRI machine consists of the primary magnet, gradient magnet, gradient coils, radiofrequency coils, radiofrequency detector, and a computer. The human body consists primarily of water (70%), which is comprised of two hydrogen and one oxygen atom held together by magnetic bonds. Each hydrogen atom has a single spinning proton; a charged proton particle produces a magnetic field referred to as a magnetic moment (Figure 3.2A). These hydrogen protons are randomly oriented until a very strong magnet is applied. The magnetic force utilized to make up the primary magnetic field in an MRI is 50,000 times stronger than the magnetic field of the Earth. When the primary magnetic field is turned on, it causes hydrogen protons to spin on an axis parallel to the magnet, like a spinning top (Figure 3.2B). Radiofrequency coils within the MRI transmit short radiofrequency waves or pulses that change the orientation of the protons. When the radiofrequency pulse is turned off or stops, it allows the proton to relax and return to its prior state of alignment with the primary magnetic field. When this occurs, energy is released in the form of radiofrequency signals; these are then read by the receiving radiofrequency coils. Gradient magnet and gradient coils all have areas of varying magnetic strength, which aid in the reading of energy exerted by the proton when applied with the radiofrequency waves. The radiofrequency coils send their received information to the radiofrequency detector; this is ultimately entered into a computer along with the information received from the gradient coils, which input the received information directly into the computer. An image is the final product (Figure 3.3).

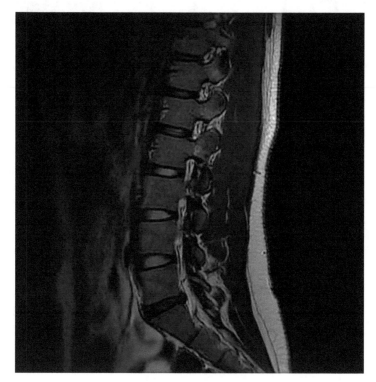

FIGURE 3.1 MR image.
Courtesy of Dr. David Begleiter.

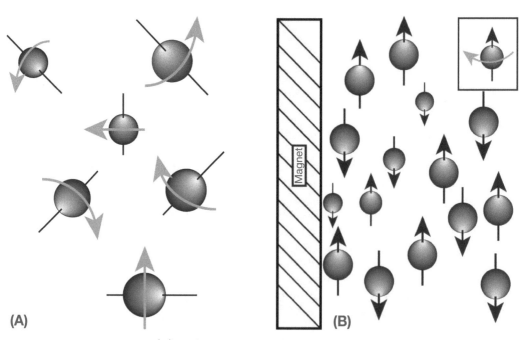

(A)   (B)

FIGURE 3.2 (A) Hydrogen atoms spinning in different directions
and (B) hydrogen atoms lined up with the magnet.
Source: Drawing by Ocean City High School student.

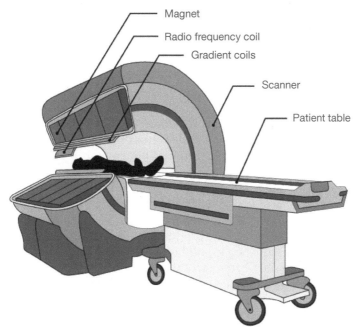

Magnet

Radio frequency coil

Gradient coils

Scanner

Patient table

FIGURE 3.3 MR scanner labeled by parts.
Source: Drawing by Ocean City High School student.

When reviewing an MR image, the energy produced by changes in the magnetic charge within body tissues is transformed by the computer into images that depict the tissue type. If tissue has little to no hydrogen, such as cortical bone or air within the lung, a dark or black area will appear on the image **(Figure 3.4)**. Conversely, if the tissue is high in hydrogen, such as in the brain, spinal column, heart, abdominal viscera and organs, and musculoskeletal system, a white area will appear on the image **(Figure 3.5)**. For this reason,

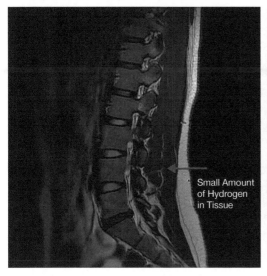

Small Amount of Hydrogen in Tissue

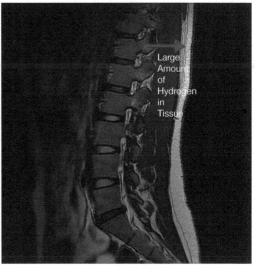

Large Amount of Hydrogen in Tissue

FIGURE 3.4 Little amount of hydrogen in tissue.
Source: Courtesy of Dr. David Begleiter; diagramming by Theresa M. Campo.

FIGURE 3.5 Large amount of hydrogen in tissue.
Source: Courtesy of Dr. David Begleiter; diagramming by Theresa M. Campo.

MR imaging is best for identifying abnormalities within these structures. MR angiography is also useful in identifying vascular abnormalities when assessing organ function. Functional MRI studies of the brain, for example, can be interpreted through changes in blood perfusion to tissue regions as seen through captured images.

The varying shades of gray are a display of pixel arrangement. Varying the sequence of radiofrequency pulses (*repetition time,* or TR) and the time between the delivery of the radiofrequency pulse and receipt of the echo signal (*time to echo,* or TE) work together to provide the image. There are two relaxation times that are recorded and produce images, they are Timi 1 (T1) and Timi 2 (T2). The longitudinal relaxation time (T1) is a constant time that determines the rate excited protons return to equilibrium, measuring the protons spinning to realign with the external magnetic field. The transverse relaxation time (T2) determines the rate excited protons reach equilibrium.

The most common sequence of images is T1 and T2 weighted scans. They are inversely proportionate, utilize short TE and TR times, and utilize T1 and T2 properties of tissue to produce either predominantly dark or bright areas on the image. FLuid-Attenuated Inversion Recovery (FLAIR) sequence is another commonly used sequence that utilizes very long TE and TR times like a T2 weighted image. Diffusion weighted imaging is very sensitive for detecting ischemia and acute stroke by detecting random movements of water protons. When water shifts from the extracellular to intracellular space from osmotic gradient during an ischemic event, it becomes restricted and this results in a very bright signal.

MRI has many uses, as discussed, and is safe during pregnancy since no ionizing radiation is used; therefore, it can detect suspected cholecystitis and appendicitis, which occur during pregnancy. Since strong magnets are used during the imaging process, patients must be screened prior to imaging for any implanted metallic substances, such as pacemakers or artificial valves or joints, to avoid displacement or complications. Automatic implantable cardioverter defibrillators (AICDs) offer a special concern as the magnet can reprogram the device; therefore, consultation with the patient's cardiologist may be required. It is also important to ascertain if patients have any known or potential retained metallic foreign bodies, especially in the eyes, brain, or other vital areas of the body that may move or shift, causing adverse complications during the study. A work history as part of the social history can aid in discovery. Since MRI studies require patients to remain still within an enclosed space for prolonged durations, it is important to assess for claustrophobia and anxiety since motion artifacts can result in an inadequate image or imaging series due to the sensitivity of the recall coils receiving information at the atomic level. Patients prone to anxiety or claustrophobia may need to be medicated prior to the test or scanned with an open MRI scanner. However, open scanners may result in poorer quality images because their magnetic strength is decreased.

Since its development and use in the 1970s, MRI has allowed for more precise and detailed imaging of the body and is safer than other modalities in that it does not utilize ionizing radiation to produce an image. As with radiographs and CT scans, contrast MRI imaging can assist in identifying different types of tissues and organs. MRI is very sensitive in differentiating soft tissue structures such as ligaments, tendons, and muscle. Because the technology uses very strong magnets, care must be given in screening patients for surgical clips, body piercings, pacemakers, and other metallic apparatus. Additionally, it is important to consider the location of objects within the external environment, such as oxygen tanks, IV poles, and so forth. MRI technology is also useful in generating detailed 3D images.

ULTRASONOGRAPHY

Ultrasonography, also known as ultrasound, has been around since its development and first use in the 1940s. Ultrasound uses sound waves to generate real-time images. It is a noninvasive method to evaluate anatomical structures and function and is also used for guiding and increasing accuracy in performing invasive procedures, such as joint aspiration and IV catheter insertion. Ultrasound can be performed at the bedside as well as in the radiology department or outpatient setting.

Ultrasound uses sound waves or pulses at a range of 1 to 17 MHz, which is well above the human's ability to hear sound, which is between 20 and 20,000 Hz. The ultrasound probe or transducer sends out and receives sound waves that are then interpreted by a computer, which generates an image in real time. The transducer transmits extremely short bursts of sound waves that can penetrate tissue. Once the sound waves reach the interface of the tissue, they return to the transducer as an echo; this echo is interpreted into an image based on the round-trip time of the pulse and echo. Once the echo arrives back to the transducer, it is converted to electrical pulses that are sent to the scanner and computer, generating an image. **Figure 3.6** demonstrates how ultrasonography works.

The final image is created by the difference between the amount of sound that is transmitted from the transducer compared with that reflected through the echo. If sound waves encounter a fluid-filled structure, most of the energy will be transmitted and appear as well-defined walls. While this may be an indication of a cyst, it is not due to the fluid nature of the cyst but rather the decreased reflection of sound or an absence of internal echo, which appears dark or black on the image. This is commonly referred to as being hypoechoic **(Figure 3.7)**. If these sound waves encounter bone or air, most of the energy is either deflected or absorbed and is seen as a bright or white shading on the image,

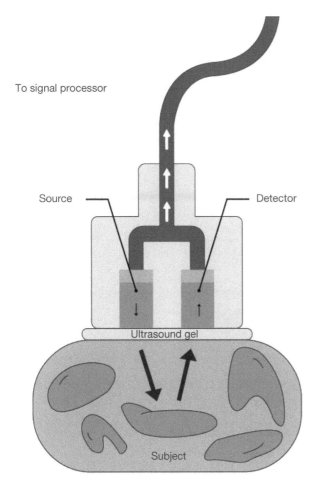

To signal processor

Source

Detector

Ultrasound gel

Subject

FIGURE 3.6 How ultrasonography works.
Source: Drawing by Ocean City High School student.

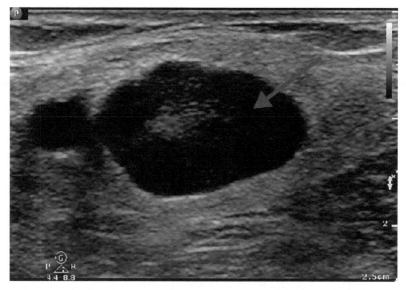

FIGURE 3.7 Fluid-filled area—hypoechoic.
Source: Theresa M. Campo/Aubrey Rybinski.

referred to as hyperechoic **(Figure 3.8)**. As with other testing modalities, there are shades and patterns between the spectrum of white and black. For example, solid tissue may have a speckled appearance with definable, visible blood vessels that appear lighter because of the hyperechoic property of vessel walls. Conversely, solid organs and fluid, which are hypoechoic, will appear darker.

Ultrasonography is performed with a patient in a comfortable position with the transducer placed on the skin against the area to be imaged. A coupling agent, consisting of a water-soluble gel or other medium, is applied to the transducer to ensure good contact and transmission of the ultrasonic waves in a controlled manner through the skin to the underlying structures. As stated earlier, transducers can produce high-frequency sound

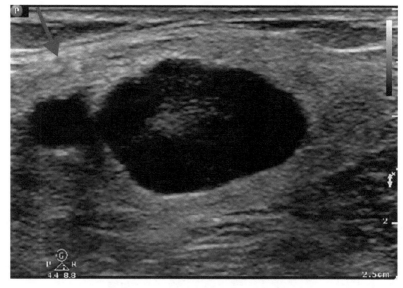

FIGURE 3.8 Air or bone—hyperechoic.
Source: Theresa M. Campo/Aubrey Rybinski.

waves between 1 and 17 MHz. Higher frequency waves produce clearer images than lower frequencies and result in less tissue penetration, making them more useful when imaging superficial structures, such as the thyroid or breasts, or when imaging infants and small children. Conversely, lower frequency waves have good tissue penetration and are best for evaluating deeper structures, such as those within the abdomen or the pelvis. However, these images lose some of their resolution.

Ultrasound images can be produced in various anatomical planes such as the axial, coronal, or sagittal planes based on the position of the transducer with regard to the position of the patient or area being studied. Transducers can also be placed inside the body, such as transvaginal, transesophageal, transrectal, or intraoral transducers, for better visualization of deep or difficult-to-see organs or structures. Since sonic waves do not readily penetrate bone or gas-filled areas, acoustic windows are used to visualize underlying structures. For example, evaluation of the liver is performed through acoustic windows in the intercostal spaces of the ribs. A transabdominal ultrasound uses the bladder to better visualize and block the air-filled colon. There are five types of ultrasounds as seen in **Table 3.1**.

Ultrasound has numerous benefits, which are increasing with advancing technology. Ultrasound provides static and dynamic real-time images, is used to increase accuracy when performing procedures, is safe to use during pregnancy and with children, and is less expensive than other testing modalities such as MRI and CT scanning. Limitations include difficulty in crossing tissue–gas and tissue–bone interfaces; in addition, image quality and interpretation are operator dependent. Therefore, it is vital that the ultrasound user become proficient in ultrasound technique for diagnostic and therapeutic purposes. There is numerous "portable" ultrasound equipment on the market for use in almost every clinical setting. The hand-held resources include a probe that can be plugged into a laptop, tablet, and even cellular phone and can be used almost everywhere.

TABLE 3.1 TYPES OF ULTRASOUND

MODE	INFORMATION
A-mode (amplitude mode)	• Simplest type • Single transducer • Spikes along a line represent the amplitude of the signal at different depths • Therapeutic scan is also done in this mode to treat tumors or calculi
B-mode (brightness mode)	• Most often used • Also known as 2D • Each echo is depicted as a dot, with thousands of dots making an image
M-mode (motion mode)	• Quick pulses in quick succession • Evaluates moving structures
Doppler	• Determines flow and velocity of blood • Shows on monitor screen as blue or red • Red indicates flow toward the transducer • Blue indicates flow away from the transducer
Duplex	• Simultaneously uses grayscale and color Doppler to visualize flow within the vessel

CONSIDERATIONS WHEN ORDERING DIAGNOSTIC MEDICAL IMAGING

When deciding on the most appropriate imaging modality to order, it is important to take into consideration how the images are obtained and what you are looking to achieve with the diagnosis. Diagnostic imaging does not replace taking a thorough history and performing a physical examination. The decision to add an imaging study must include consideration of risks and benefits, cost to the patient as well as to the institution, and potential adverse effects (e.g., anaphylaxis, teratogenic harm during pregnancy). Collaboration with colleagues, including radiologists and radiology technologists, is key to achieving appropriate care of the patient and identification of problems or potential problems.

Resources to improve decision-making in diagnostic imaging include use of the American College of Radiology (ACR) Appropriateness Criteria, which are evidence-based and regularly updated. These guidelines and algorithms are organized by symptom and suspected condition and aid in decision-making.

The ACR Appropriateness Criteria provide quality ratings for various medical imaging studies based on complaint or working diagnosis. For example, if a pulmonary embolus is suspected, a list of radiological studies is given with ratings, comments, and the relative radiation level. Rating scales range from 1 to 9, with 1 to 3 being "usually not appropriate," 4 to 6 "may be appropriate," and 7 to 9 "usually appropriate."

CONCLUSION

MRI and ultrasound, although different in how they produce physical images, are similar in safety since neither involves exposure to ionizing radiation. MRI has many advantages, including the contrast of images and the ability to reconstruct images for enhanced detail. Disadvantages include cost, time to complete the study, and potential complications from implanted metallic medical devices. In addition, some patients may not be able to tolerate the restrictions imposed during testing.

The benefits of ultrasound include cost, safety, portable access, and real-time imaging, making diagnosis and therapeutic interventions much easier. Limitations include image quality that is highly operator dependent and difficult to obtain in the morbidly obese individual or when imagining structures through bone and air/gas. However, its use is increasing with smaller, more digitally enhanced machines.

RESOURCES

American College of Radiology. (n.d.). *Appropriateness criteria.* http://www.acr.org/quality-safety/appropriateness-criteria

Au-Yong, I., Au-Yong, A., & Broderick, N. (2010). *On-call x-rays made easy.* Churchill Livingstone, Elsevier.

Brant, W. E. (2012a). Abdomen ultrasound. In W. E. Brant & C. A. Helms (Eds.), *Fundamentals of diagnostic radiology* (4th ed., pp. 858–885). Wolters Kluwer/Lippincott Williams & Wilkins.

Brant, W. E. (2012b). Chest, thyroid, parathyroid, and neonatal brain. In W. E. Brant & C. A. Helms (Eds.), *Fundamentals of diagnostic radiology* (4th ed., pp. 936–953). Wolters Kluwer/Lippincott Williams & Wilkins.

Brant, W. E. (2012c). Diagnostic imaging methods. In W. E. Brant & C. A. Helms (Eds.), *Fundamentals of diagnostic radiology* (4th ed., pp. 2–27). Wolters Kluwer/Lippincott Williams & Wilkins.

Brant, W. E. (2012d). Genital tract and bladder ultrasound. In W. E. Brant & C. A. Helms (Eds.), *Fundamentals of diagnostic radiology* (4th ed., pp. 886–909). Wolters Kluwer/ Lippincott Williams & Wilkins.

Brant, W. E., & Dougherty, R. S. (2012). Vascular ultrasound. In W. E. Brant & C. A. Helms (Eds.), *Fundamentals of diagnostic radiology* (4th ed., pp. 954–979). Wolters Kluwer/ Lippincott Williams & Wilkins.

Currie, S., Hoggard, N., Craven, I. J., Hadjivassiliou, M., &Wilkinson, I. D. (2013). Understanding MRI: Basic MR physics for physicians. *Postgraduate Medical Journal, 89,* 209–223. https://doi.org/10.1136/postgradmedj-2012-131342

Daffner, R. H. (2014). Overview and principles of diagnostic imaging. In R. H. Daffner & M. S. Hartman (Eds.), *Clinical radiology: The essentials* (4th ed., pp. 1–42). Wolters Kluwer/ Lippincott Williams & Wilkins.

Daffner, R. H., & Hartman, R. H. (2014). Radiographic contrast agents. In R. H. Daffner & M. S. Hartman (Eds.), *Clinical radiology: The essentials* (4th ed., pp. 43–48). Wolters Kluwer/Lippincott Williams & Wilkins.

Herring, W. (2016). *Learning radiology: Recognizing the* basics (3rd ed., pp. 1–7, 204–227). Elsevier.

Preston, D. C. (2016). *Magnetic resonance imaging (MRI) of the brain and spine: Basics.* https:// case.edu/med/neurology/NR/MRI%20Basics.htm

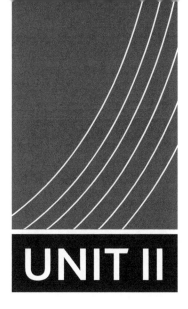

UNIT II

Interpreting Chest and Abdominal Radiographs

CHAPTER 4

Basic Interpretation of the Chest

► VIDEOS

4.1: Introduction
4.2: Interpretation of the Chest—Normal

Accompanying videos can be accessed online at https://connect.springerpub
.com/content/book/978-0-8261-6047-8/chapter/ch04

The interpretation of chest radiographs can be gratifying as well as frustrating. It may take many years of experience looking at radiographs to gain competency and confidence in interpretation. However, we all must start somewhere, so this chapter is meant to introduce you to the basic interpretation of chest radiographs. This chapter includes a brief review of the radiographic densities discussed earlier in this book, adequacy of radiographs and why this is important, and pediatric considerations. It is important to understand what you are looking at so you can identify not only normal structures but also abnormal findings. Plain radiographs are excellent in evaluating normal structures of the chest, foreign bodies, and gross abnormalities within the chest and surrounding structures that may lead to further radiological evaluation.

RADIOGRAPHIC DENSITIES

Radiographic density refers to the degree of blackness of the film. It allows for radiographic contrast, and therefore provides the ability to differentiate various structures (Figure 4.1). Structures with high physical density produce less radiodensity and vice versa. When a structure has a low radiodensity, the rays easily penetrate the structure, resulting in low absorbency; this causes blackening of the film. When a structure has a high radiodensity, the passage of rays is impeded; in other words, there is high absorbency. This results in a bright or white appearance on the film. Structures with varying degrees of radiodensity and absorption or attenuation give varying shades of gray within the spectrum of black and white. Contrast between adjacent structures is increased when there is a difference in radiodensity or thickness of those structures. Whether evaluating the structures of the chest, abdomen, spine, or extremities, this black-and-white spectrum is important in understanding exactly what you are visualizing on the radiographs. Figure 4.1 demonstrates these concepts.

ADEQUACY OF RADIOGRAPHS

Image quality is paramount to accurately review and identify normal and abnormal findings on radiographs. Image quality can be affected by motion, scatter, magnification, thickness, and distortion, as discussed in Chapter 2 of this text. When reviewing radiographs, remember that the body is three-dimensional; however, radiographs produce two-dimensional images using shades of gray that depict structures of varying densities. It is also important to have a firm recollection and understanding of basic anatomy and physiology. When

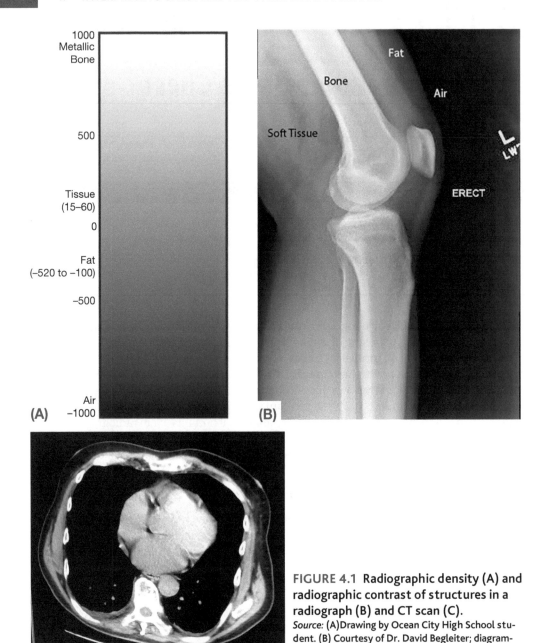

FIGURE 4.1 Radiographic density (A) and radiographic contrast of structures in a radiograph (B) and CT scan (C).
Source: (A)Drawing by Ocean City High School student. (B) Courtesy of Dr. David Begleiter; diagramming by Theresa M. Campo. (C) Courtesy of Theresa M. Campo.

discussing, reporting, and documenting findings of the chest x-ray, remember that these are findings and not diagnoses. Stating that you visualize a patchy infiltrate of the right middle lobe is a finding. However, stating that you visualize a right middle lobe pneumonia is not correct because a diagnosis results from a synthesis of a thorough health history and physical examination findings, along with the finding of a patchy infiltrate in the right middle lobe.

As with anything in medicine and nursing, there are rules in place to help not only guide the interpretation of radiographs, but also to help avoid missing findings or having false negatives and false positives. It is important that you "treat the patient" and not the radiographs. This is accomplished through a comprehensive and thorough health history and physical examination prior to ordering the diagnostic study. Any diagnostic imaging study should only be ordered if it will add to the diagnosis and subsequent treatment of a suspected condition, whether a plain radiograph, CT scan, MRI, or other modality. It is imperative that providers reduce a patient's risk of unnecessary and repeated radiation exposure and its dire consequences. Additionally, when ordering a radiograph, the entire image must be carefully and systematically studied in the same manner every single time. This will help to avoid missed findings or making an interpretation based on an assumption rather than a thorough evaluation of the image. If a finding is identified on a radiograph that is inconsistent with the patient's initial examination, one must go back and reevaluate that patient to identify whether the finding on the image is an incidental finding or related to the initial complaint.

As stated earlier, radiographs are taken in a single view. For this reason, it is important to obtain at least two views of an area requiring evaluation. If the patient were to hold an object in front of their body with the x-ray taken from either front to back or back to front, one may not be able to visualize the object in those views. However, if the image were taken from a lateral view—from the patient's side—then the object would be visualized easily. Conversely, if the patient held objects in their hands with arms held straight out and the image taken laterally, the objects may not be readily seen. However, an anterior or posterior view would provide an image of the laterally held objects. It is also important to compare current with previous studies to ascertain changes over time as well as to confirm normal anatomy for that individual. When evaluating extremities, comparison views can be very helpful, especially in pediatric patients, to identify whether a finding is abnormal or normal. To ensure quality and safety in diagnostic interpretation, all radiographs should be reviewed by experienced and trained radiologists in addition to the provider who is evaluating the patient. Continued collaboration with radiologists and radiology technicians, as well as colleagues, is imperative for quality care of all patients.

Before interpretation of a chest x-ray begins, the patient's name, date, and correct study must be confirmed. Once confirmation is complete, then determination of adequacy of the film must be done. Position, inspiration, penetration, and rotation need to be considered in order to deem a study to be adequate. The direction that the beam travels through the patient and the cassette determines the title of the position. When the patient is facing the cartridge with the x-ray machine behind them, the image is labeled posterior–anterior (PA); conversely, if the cartridge is behind the patient with the machine in front of them, the image is labeled anterior–posterior (AP; **Figure 4.2**). The PA view is most often performed for optimal evaluation of the chest. The heart and mediastinum sit more anteriorly in the chest;

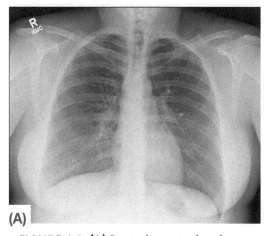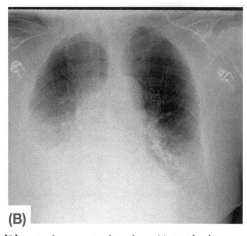

(A)   (B)

FIGURE 4.2 (A) Posterior–anterior view versus **(B)** anterior–posterior view. Note the hazy borders of landmarks, large heart, widened aorta, and white appearance of the film, overall.
Source: Courtesy of Dr. David Begleiter.

when imaged in this view, they are truer to size. The AP view is usually done as a portable image. When the rays travel from the front to the back of the person, magnification occurs; this causes the heart and mediastinum to appear bigger in size and are not seen as clearly.

A lateral view image is when the patient is standing between the cassette and the x-ray machine and the beam is traveling right to left **(Figure 4.3)**. The lateral decubitus view image requires that the patient lie on their side for 3 to 5 minutes before the frontal view is taken. This allows any fluid to settle and air to rise, which may demonstrate free air or fluid abnormalities **(Figure 4.4)**. All films should be marked left or right along with the view. For example, if an AP view is taken and not labeled, it may be assumed that it is a PA view, leading to a false reading that results from normal differences of the two views. In a normal PA view, the lung markings are more distinct, the heart is smaller, the clavicles are superimposed over the upper lung fields, and the cervical and thoracic vertebrae are more clearly visible **(Figure 4.5)**. However, in the AP view, the heart appears larger than normal with shallow lung volumes and higher sitting clavicles **(Figure 4.6)**.

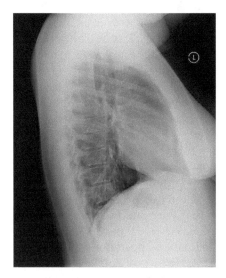

FIGURE 4.3 Lateral view.
Source: Courtesy of Theresa M. Campo.

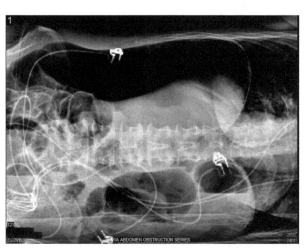

FIGURE 4.4 Lateral decubitus view.
Source: Courtesy of Theresa M. Campo.

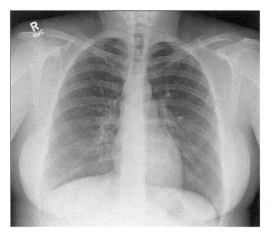

FIGURE 4.5 Posterior–anterior chest.
Source: Courtesy of Dr. David Begleiter.

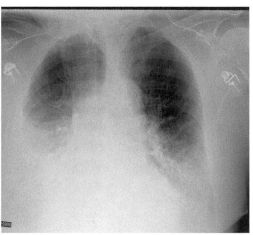

FIGURE 4.6 Anterior–posterior chest.
Source: Courtesy of Theresa M. Campo.

During any chest radiographic imaging, the patient will be asked to take a deep breath and hold it. This allows for better visualization of the structures within and around the chest cavity. Normal inspiration is determined by counting the anterior and posterior ribs. The diaphragm should cross the level of the 10th posterior rib; however, if it is between the eighth and 10th posterior ribs or at the level of the fifth or sixth anterior ribs, the image is acceptable. One would think that the ribs appearing closest to the person viewing the film are the anterior ribs. However, they are the posterior ribs (Figure 4.7). Recall the normal anatomy of the thorax. If there is a poor inspiratory effort, the film may not be accurately evaluated, as demonstrated in Figure 4.8. Counting the ribs visualized over the lung on a plain radiograph can help indicate if there were adequate inspiration. A chest radiograph may also be performed during expiration. This method is used to evaluate a patient for either pneumothorax or foreign body in the bronchus. During expiration, a foreign body in the bronchus may cause a shift in the mediastinum and heart due to the lack of volume in the affected side. Similarly, during expiration, you may see enlargement of a pneumothorax, making it more visible.

Differences in physical density impact the penetration and absorption of x-rays. If structures are not properly penetrated, there will be poor film quality with clarity and shifts in the shades of gray spectrum. The same radiation dose cannot be used for all patients since body size will affect ray penetration; this can result in over- or underexposed images negatively affecting the adequacy of the film.

Normally, in the PA view, you should be able to visualize the thoracic spine through the heart shadow and be able to see the intravertebral discs of the upper cervical spine (Figure 4.9). Underpenetration can cause an image to be too light; if this happens, the thoracic spine will not be visible through the heart shadow (Figure 4.10). Additionally, the hemidiaphragm may not be visible and consequently may be mistaken for a left lower lobe

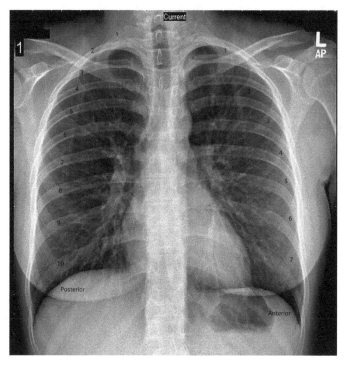

FIGURE 4.7 Inspiration with proper number of ribs.
Source: Courtesy of Dr. David Begleiter.

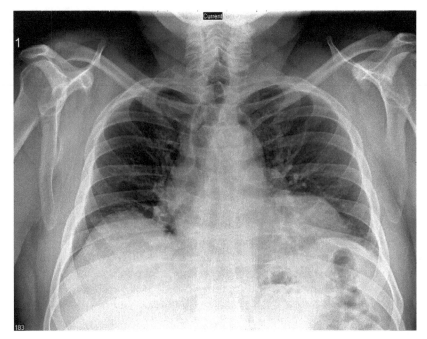

**FIGURE 4.8 Poor inspiration. Note the height of the
diaphragms and distortion of structures.**
Source: Courtesy of Dr. David Begleiter.

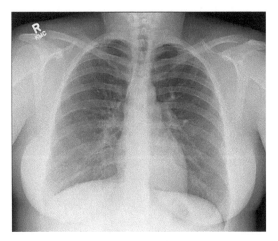

**FIGURE 4.9 Normal chest posterior–
anterior view.**
Source: Courtesy of Dr. David Begleiter.

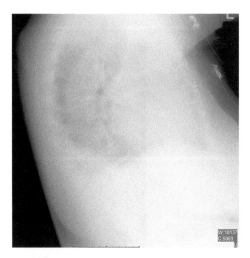

FIGURE 4.10 Underpenetration.
Source: Courtesy of Dr. David Begleiter.

infiltrate, consolidation, or pleural effusion. When an image is overpenetrated, it appears dark with decreased or loss of lung markings that can be mistaken for emphysema or a pneumothorax (**Figure 4.11**).

Finally, rotation can also have a negative effect on film adequacy. Distortion of normal anatomical structures can occur when a patient is rotated (**Figure 4.12**). It is important that patients stand parallel to the cassette with shoulders back, taking a deep breath and holding it. If the person has one shoulder in front of the other, this can cause rotation and inadequacy of that image. The heads of the clavicle, ribs, and spinal processes should be symmetrical and at equal heights bilaterally. A trick to determining rotation is to look at the medial aspects of the clavicles in relation to the spinal processes to ensure that they are of equal height and appear equally spaced from one side to the other.

Once adequacy has been determined and accepted, then the interpretation of the film can begin. When interpreting any radiographs, it is important to remember the *ABCDEs*: : *A*dequacy/*A*irway, *B*reathing or *B*irdcages, *C*ardiac/*C*irculation, *D*iaphragm, *E*dges, and *s*keleton/*s*oft tissue.

We have already discussed the adequacy of the film and now we are going to discuss the other *A*, which is *A*irway. The trachea should be midline and seen all the way to the carina (tracheal bifurcation) at the approximate level of the T4 to T5 **(Figure 4.13)**. The trachea

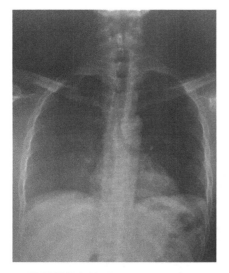

FIGURE 4.11 Overpenetration.
Source: Courtesy of Dr. Keith Lafferty.

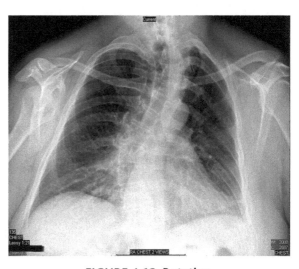

FIGURE 4.12 Rotation.
Source: Courtesy of Dr. David Begleiter.

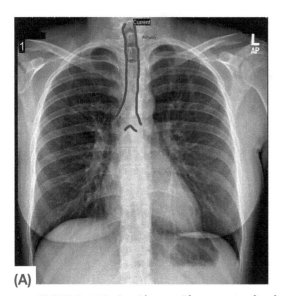

(A)

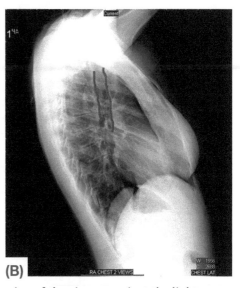

(B)

FIGURE 4.13 A = Airway. Please note the darkening of the airway against the lighter
wall. In (A) you should visualize the trachea to the carina (bifurcation);
in (B) you can also visualize the airway.
Source: Courtesy of Dr. David Begleiter; diagramming by Theresa M. Campo.

is an air-filled tube, so they should have a dark appearance because they are surrounded by soft tissue, which is lighter in color and allows for contrast. The trachea should angle downward to the thoracic inlet and be identifiable by the retrotracheal line, which should not exceed 3 mm. One can visualize the structures because they are surrounded by soft tissue, which appears lighter, giving a contrasting appearance. If there is thickening of the outlining of the airway, then it is labeled a bronchogram. A bronchogram is made visible by the surrounding alveoli containing fluid or exudate such as mucus. A bronchogram can be diagnostic for neoplasm, severe interstitial disease, pulmonary edema, consolidation, or nonobstructive pulmonary atelectasis. However, a bronchogram in some individuals may be normal and not a sign of pathology (Figure 4.14).

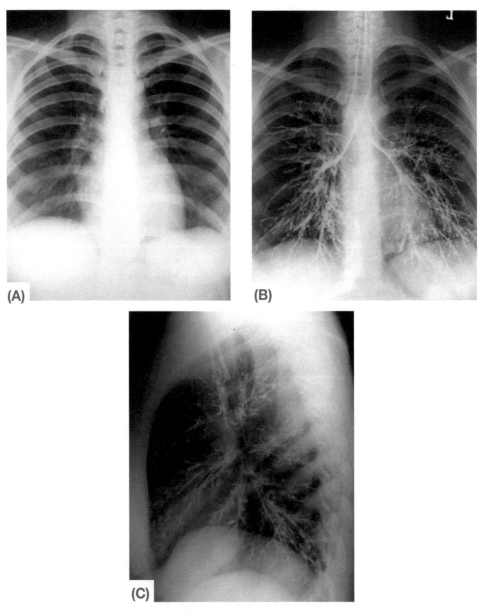

(A)   (B)

(C)

FIGURE 4.14 Bronchogram: (A) demonstrates a bronchogram on plain radiograph; (B) and (C) demonstrate a contrasted radiograph.
Source: Courtesy of Associate Professor Frank Gaillard, Radiopaedia.org.

When evaluating the *B* of our *ABCDEs* mnemonic, we think about *B*reathing. I like to evaluate this by looking at the *B*irdcages (**Figure 4.15**). If you look at the area on each side of the pleural cavity encasing the lungs, they have the appearance of a birdcage. You want to evaluate both birdcages and note whether they are comparable in appearance. You should be able to visualize the pleural tissue filling both birdcages. If you notice a brighter or whiter area in one birdcage that is not in the other, then you need to identify the finding as an abnormality. This is when knowledge of basic anatomy is key in identifying normal structures and abnormalities within the birdcage.

Each lung lobe has anatomical segments that are supplied by their own bronchus and blood vessels. The right lung has three lobes—the upper, middle, and lower; the left has two lobes—the upper and lower. The segments of the right upper lobe are the apical, anterior, and posterior segments. The middle lobe includes the medial and lateral segments. The lower lobe has the most segments and includes the superior, posterior, medial, anterior, and lateral base segments. The left upper lobe has a fused apical–posterior segment, as well as anterior, superior, and inferior segments. The left lower lobe is like the right lower lobe except the anterior and medial basal segments are fused.

The pleura is made up of two layers: the visceral and parietal layers. The visceral layer covers the lung and is not readily visualized on radiographs. However, it may be normal to visualize the interlobar fissures. There are two interlobar fissures on the right: the oblique, or major, and the horizontal, or minor. The left interlobar fissure consists of only the oblique fissure. The oblique fissures are normally at the level of T4 and extend downward, ending at the anterior sixth rib. The horizontal fissure begins at the level of the sixth rib and then extends laterally and anteriorly downward to the medial section of the fourth rib.

The center of the chest is where we look for our *C*, which represents the *C*ardiac silhouette and *C*irculation (**Figure 4.16**). Note that the heart silhouette sits in the center, slightly to the left. At the superior aspect of the heart, you will notice the aorta, which should be small and not enlarged or tortuous. You will also notice the branches of a tree coming out into each of our birdcages, which is the pulmonary vasculature. The heart silhouette should be less than half the width of the chest cavity. One would expect the tracings in the birdcage to be the bronchi, but they are the pulmonary vasculature. The bronchi are air filled and

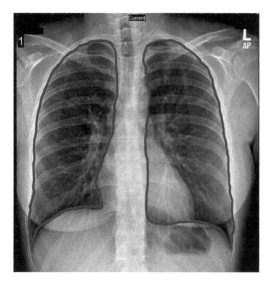

FIGURE 4.15 B = Breathing/Birdcages.
Source: Courtesy of Dr. David Begleiter; diagramming by Theresa M. Campo.

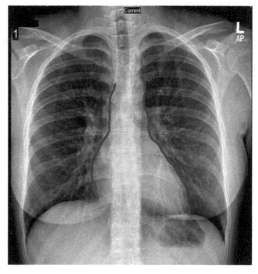

FIGURE 4.16 C = Cardiac/circulation.
Source: Courtesy of Dr. David Begleiter; diagramming by Theresa M. Campo.

hidden by the air in the lungs, which obscures them due to the similar density. One can visualize the vasculature because it is fluid filled against the air-filled lungs and bronchi, allowing for contrast and visualization. If the heart silhouette goes beyond the midline, then it is enlarged; the cardiothoracic ratio should be roughly 1:2.

Our *D*iaphragms represent the *D* of our *ABCDEs mnemonic*. The right hemidiaphragm sits higher than the left hemidiaphragm due to the contiguity of the left ventricle of the heart with the left diaphragm, not because of the bulk or size of the liver (Figure 4.17). When both diaphragms sit at the same level, it can be due to normal physiologic reasons, such as with pregnancy, which can push up the left hemidiaphragm, or from pathologic causes such as diaphragmatic rupture or other trauma. Emphysema can cause blunting of the costophrenic angles at the lateral aspect of the diaphragm because of excessive air trapping. Additionally, the hyperinflation of chronic obstructive pulmonary disease (COPD) can cause the hemidiaphragms to appear level with each other.

The *E* is for *E*dges. What you want to do here is look at the edges of your birdcage and its contents to see that the edges are crisp and clearly visualized (Figure 4.18). If you notice hazing or blurring of any of these edges, it may indicate an abnormality. For example, blurring or hazing indicating an increased density over the right diaphragm may be suggestive of a right lower lobe infiltrate or consolidation.

Finally, we need to evaluate *s*—the *s*keleton and *s*oft tissue outside the chest cavity. These are important areas to evaluate for fractures, neoplasm, free air, and foreign bodies. Again, it is imperative that you evaluate the entire radiograph left to right and top to bottom, including everything in between. The lower cervical (pointing down) and thoracic vertebrae (pointing up), ribs, clavicles, scapula, humeral heads, and the sternum (lateral view only) should all be visualized on the chest radiograph. The radiograph should also include identifiable patient information, the date, and technologist markers, as well as the type of study being done. Within this age of digital technology, the identifiable patient demographic information, as well as the type of study, reason for this study, and ordering provider, may be separate from the image itself (Figure 4.19).

The *ABCDEs* criteria are used when evaluating radiographs to allow providers to identify normal from abnormal findings. Discussion of the type of abnormal findings that can

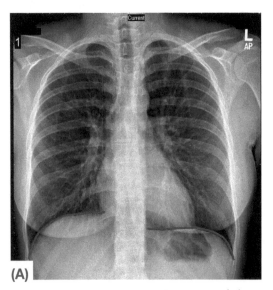 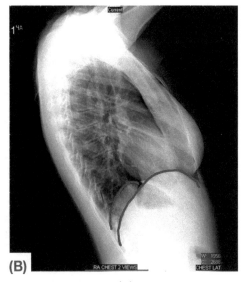

(A)   (B)

FIGURE 4.17 D = Diaphragms on (A) posterior–anterior view and (B) lateral view.
Source: Courtesy of Dr. David Begleiter; diagramming by Theresa M. Campo.

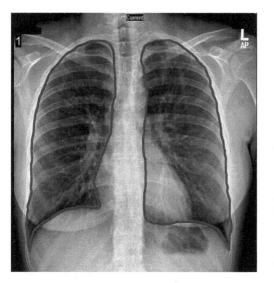

FIGURE 4.18 E = Edges.
Source: Courtesy of Dr. David Begleiter; diagramming by Theresa M. Campo.

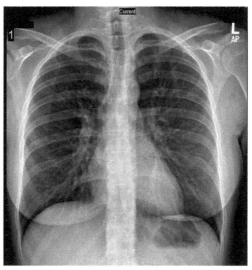

FIGURE 4.19 S = Skeletal/Soft tissue.
Source: Courtesy of Dr. David Begleiter.

be visualized on a radiograph is discussed in Chapter 5. The ability to identify what is occurring in a pathologic process will assist in anticipating and visualizing findings on radiographs. For example, pathology of the air spaces may be identified as consolidation or atelectasis because the normally air-filled areas are either fluid filled or the walls have collapsed. Fluid accumulation in the pleural space is identified as an effusion, emphysema and asthma may result from overinflation of the lungs, and interstitial changes may be from fibrosis and/or edema. Over time, with practice in viewing multiple chest radiographs, differentiating normal from abnormal findings will only get easier and you will begin to feel more confident reviewing and documenting findings. I guarantee you'll enjoy the process as you get more proficient and comfortable with your interpretations.

PEDIATRIC CONSIDERATIONS (COMPARISON OF ADULT AND INFANT/CHILD X-RAYS)

Interpreting chest x-rays of infants and children can be challenging. Normal anatomical structures in adults may look completely different in children and not be considered abnormal. Anatomical structures change with growth as children become older. Obtaining an adequate film on infants and children may also be challenging due to lack of cooperation or inability to follow commands.

In infants and small children, the heart may appear larger in size and take up much of the chest cavity, making it difficult to visualize the pulmonary vasculature and pleura (Figure 4.20). The thymus may cause confusion and be mistaken for a mass in the upper chest in pediatric chest radiographs because it is readily visualized in infants and small children. However, as a child grows, the thymus remains the same size and eventually becomes obscured and not visible in adult patient images. When viewing the skeleton of pediatric patients, the bones may not be as bright or white as in adults because pediatric bone is more fibrous and not as calcified as mature bone which has higher levels of calcium. Children also have growth plates at the epiphyseal regions of bones that may appear as fractures or breaks in the bony cortex, but these are normal ossification centers and are discussed in detail in the extremity chapters.

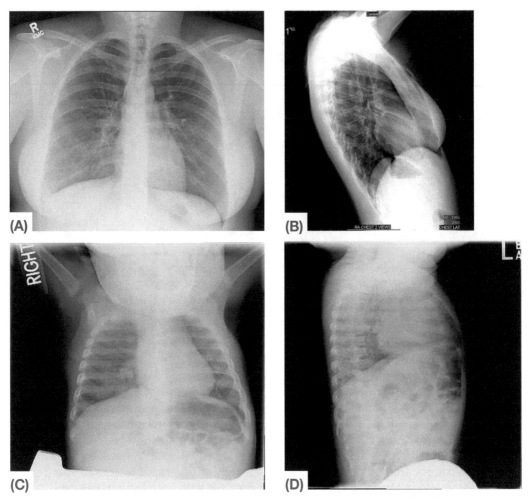

FIGURE 4.20 Comparing child and adult chest x-rays: (A) Normal adult chest x-ray and (B) normal adult chest x-ray lateral. (C) Normal child chest x-ray and (D) normal child chest x-ray lateral.
Source: Courtesy of Dr. David Begleiter.

MEDIASTINAL WIDTH

The mediastinum is the central thorax between the lungs and the heart and is divided into three regions: the anterior, middle, and posterior regions.

Anterior—area behind the sternum and in front of the heart and great vessels

Middle—area between the anterior and posterior pericardium that includes the pericardium, heart, aortic arch, proximal brachialcephalic vessels, pulmonary veins and arteries, trachea and main bronchi, and lymph nodes

Posterior—area behind the heart and trachea that includes the vertebral bodies

Some literature also includes the superior region that is above the heart and great vessels. The aorta should be small and tight and not tortuous or widened (Figure 4.21). If the aorta is wide in appearance, the first thing that must be done is make sure the film is

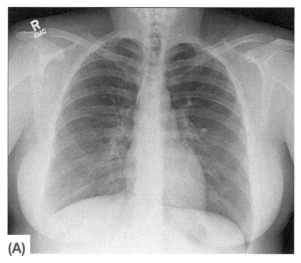
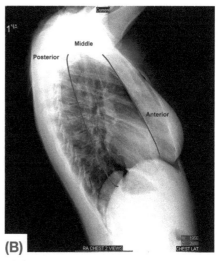

FIGURE 4.21 (A) Normal mediastinal width; (B) widened mediastinum.
Source: Courtesy of Dr. David Begleiter; diagramming by Theresa M. Campo.

adequate and that you are looking at the proper view. If everything is acceptable, then consideration for a CT scan should be the next step to further evaluate the aorta and mediastinum for abnormalities.

CONCLUSION

This chapter introduced the reader to examining chest films. Chest radiograph interpretation can be intimidating, but once you are used to the geography of the chest, identification of normal and abnormal findings fall into place. Take each image one at a time, collaborate with colleagues and radiologists, and look at as many images as you can. One recommendation I give students is to look at the study and then read the radiologist's interpretation and compare. If the radiologist comments on something, look for it, so you will be familiar with that finding the next time you see it.

RESOURCES

Au-Yong, I., Au-Yong, A., & Broderick, N. (2010). *On-call x-rays made easy.* Churchill Livingstone, Elsevier.

Collins, J., & Stern, E. J. (2008). *Chest radiology: The essentials* (2nd ed.). Wolters Kluwer/ Lippincott Williams & Wilkins.

Gay, S. B., Olazagasti, J., Higginbotham, J. W., Gupta, A., Wurm, A., & Nguyen, J. (n.d.). *Introduction to chest radiology.* https://www.med-ed.virginia.edu/courses/rad/cxr /Index.html

Goodman, L. R. (2015). *Felson's principles of chest roentgenology: A programmed text* (4th ed.). Elsevier Saunders.

Herring, W. (2016). *learning radiology: Recognizing the basics* (3rd ed., pp. 8–34). Elsevier.

John, S. D., & Swischuk, L. E. (2012). Pediatric chest. In W. E. Brant & C. A. Helms (Eds.), *Fundamentals of diagnostic radiology* (4th ed., pp. 1128–1175). Wolters Kluwer/Lippincott Williams & Wilkins.

Klein, J. S. (2012). Mediastinum and hila. In W. E. Brant & C. A. Helms (Eds.), *Fundamentals of diagnostic radiology* (4th ed., pp. 367–396). Wolters Kluwer/Lippincott Williams & Wilkins.

Lemo, J., & Klein, J. S. (2012). Methods of examination, normal anatomy, and radiographic findings of chest disease. In W. E. Brant & C. A. Helms (Eds.), *Fundamentals of diagnostic radiology* (4th ed., pp. 324–366). Wolters Kluwer/Lippincott.

Mueller, J. S., & Daffner, R. H. (2014). Cardiac imaging. In R. H. Daffner & M. S. Hartman (Eds.), *Clinical radiology: The essentials* (4th ed., pp. 163–202). Wolters Kluwer/Lippincott Williams & Wilkins.

Mueller, J. S., & Daffner, R. H. (2014). Chest imaging. In R. H. Daffner & M. S. Hartman (Eds.), *Clinical radiology: The essentials* (4th ed., pp. 79–162). Wolters Kluwer/Lippincott Williams & Wilkins.

Shelton, D. K. (2012). Cardiac anatomy, physiology, and imaging modalities. In W. E. Brant & C. A. Helms (Eds.), *Fundamentals of diagnostic radiology* (4th ed., pp. 568–594). Wolters Kluwer/Lippincott Williams & Wilkins.

CHAPTER 5

Abnormalities Found on Radiographs of the Chest

► VIDEOS

5.1: Interpretation of the Chest—Density Abnormalities
5.2: Interpretation of the Chest—Air Abnormalities

Accompanying videos can be accessed online at https://connect.springerpub
.com/content/book/978-0-8261-6047-8/chapter/ch05

There are many abnormalities that can be identified on a chest radiograph. The intent of this chapter is to introduce some of the more common findings seen on a chest radiograph including atelectasis, pulmonary edema, pleural effusion, a consolidation, pneumothorax, tension pneumothorax, pneumomediastinum, hyperaeration, SARS-COV-2 (COVID-19), and masses and tumors. The more radiographs you review and evaluate, the more findings of normal variants and abnormalities you will be able to identify.

ATELECTASIS

Atelectasis is a condition of volume loss in a portion of the lung involving a subsegment, segment, lobe, or the entire lung. Atelectasis appears as a dense or lighter area on the x-ray that is usually linear but may also have a curvilinear or wedge-shaped appearance on film. Atelectasis most commonly occurs from obstruction, usually of the bronchus by a mucous plug, neoplasm, or a foreign body. It may also be compressive and caused by a tumor, heart enlargement, hypoinflation, or emphysematous bullae. Patients who have had granulomatous diseases such as tuberculosis, pulmonary infarct, or trauma may have scar tissue that can also cause atelectasis. It can be adhesive from the inactivation of surfactant, or passive with the normal compliance of the lung within the pneumothorax or pleural effusion when the airway remains patent. Atelectasis may be present in one lobe or in multiple lobes. Because of the volume loss of air in the affected area, the findings on radiographs will be brighter/lighter shades of gray within the birdcage (Figure 5.1).

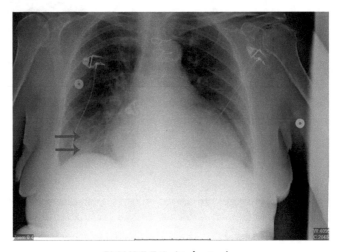

FIGURE 5.1 **Atelectasis.**
Source: Courtesy of Theresa M. Campo.

PULMONARY EDEMA

There are two basic types of pulmonary edema: cardiogenic and noncardiogenic. Cardiogenic pulmonary edema is caused by increased hydrostatic pulmonary capillary pressure, whereas noncardiogenic pulmonary edema is caused by an alteration in capillary membrane permeability or decreased plasma oncotic pressure. So just think of this simplistically: Cardiogenic edema is failure of the pump, whereas noncardiogenic edema is a problem with the plumbing and associated structures leading to or from the heart.

Pulmonary edema may result in a variety of patterns on a plain radiograph of the chest. These include cephalization of the pulmonary vessels, Kerly A lines, Kerly B lines, peribronchial cuffing, bat wing pattern, patchy shadowing with an air bronchogram, heart enlargement, and/or pleural effusions **(Figure 5.2)**.

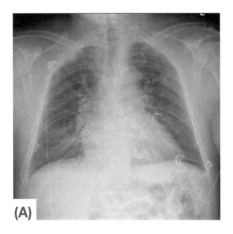

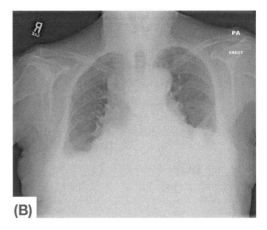

(A)   (B)

FIGURE 5.2 (A) Pulmonary edema; (B) pulmonary edema with pleural effusion cardiomegaly with mediastinum widening;

(continued)

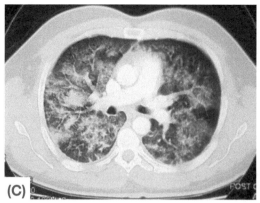

(C)

FIGURE 5.2 (*continued*)
(C) CT scan axial view contrast-enhanced demonstrating alveolar and interstitial pulmonary edema.
Source: (A, B) Courtesy of Dr. Frank Gaillard, Radiopaedia. org. (C) Reproduced with permission from Medscape Drugs & Diseases (https://emedicine.medscape. com/), Noncardiogenic Pulmonary Edema Imaging, 2018, available at: https://emedicine.medscape.com/article/360932-overview.

PLEURAL EFFUSION

Pleural effusions may be caused by congestive heart failure, infection, trauma, pulmonary embolus, tumor, autoimmune disease, ascites, and/or renal failure. Regardless of the cause, it is important to identify a pleural effusion and make the decision, based on clinical and diagnostic findings, whether the effusion needs to be treated. Pleural effusions are collections of fluid in the pleural space and can be identified using plain radiographs, but they may also be identified and further evaluated with CT scan and ultrasonography. On plain films they will often appear as a meniscus or straight line.

On an upright posterior–anterior (PA) image, blunting of the costophrenic angle(s) will be seen with a pleural effusion as fluid settles in the lowest or most dependent regions, which are the costophrenic angles. If a lateral decubitus image is obtained, identification of a pleural effusion can be made similarly by looking at a tabletop appearance of the affected lung. Large effusions can cause the mediastinum to shift away from the side of the effusion **(Figure 5.3)**.

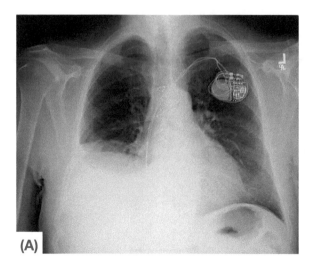

(A)

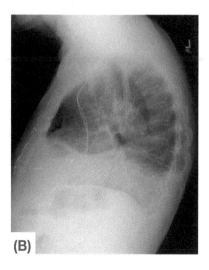

(B)

FIGURE 5.3 (A, B) Pleural effusion. Note the loss of the lower right birdcage especially the costophrenic angle.

(*continued*)

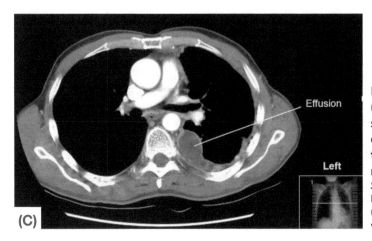

FIGURE 5.3 (*continued*) (C) CT scan of chest showing loculated pleural effusion in left side. Some thickening of pleura is also noted.
Source: (A, B) Courtesy of Dr. David Begleiter; (C) courtesy Drriad (https://commons.wikimedia.org/wiki/File:Pleura_effusion.jpg).

INTERPRETATION OF INFILTRATES AND CONSOLIDATION

Infiltrates and consolidations are representative of opacities that are seen as bright or lighter gray to white on an image. What is important to know is the location of the opacity to identify the location of the abnormality. When we discussed the ABCs (*a*dequacy/*a*irway, *b*reathing or *b*irdcages, *c*ardiac/*c*irculation) of interpretation of the chest film, we evaluated the edges within our birdcages. The right heart border is adjacent to the right middle lobe and the right diaphragm is representative of the right lower lobe. The left heart border is adjacent to the left upper lobe and the left diaphragm to the left lower lobe **(Figure 5.4)**. The lingula is visualized over the heart shadow on the AP or PA view. If these edges are not crisp and clear but are hazy or not identifiable, then you are visualizing an infiltrate or consolidation, which may represent a pneumonia, pneumonitis, or mass **(Figure 5.5)**. If an opacity

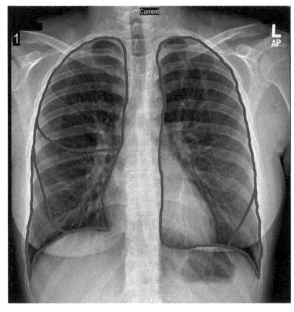

FIGURE 5.4 Chest x-ray with lobe borders.
Source: Courtesy of Dr. David Begleiter; diagramming by Theresa M. Campo.

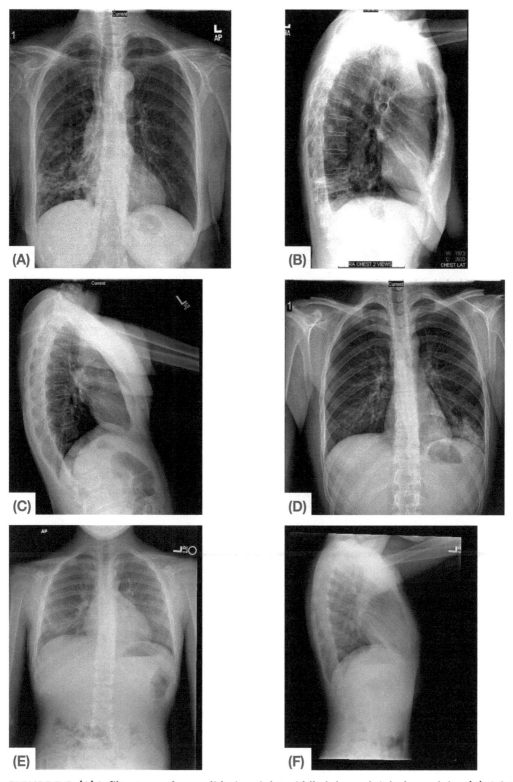

FIGURE 5.5 (A) Infiltrates and consolidation right middle lobe and right lower lobe; (B) right middle lobe and right lower lobe lateral view; (C) normal triangle behind heart silhouette; (D) left lower lobe; (E) right middle lobe; (F) right middle lobe lateral view.

(continued)

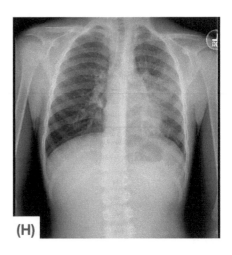

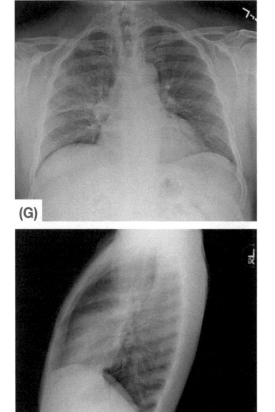

FIGURE 5.5 (continued)
(G) Anterior segment right upper
lobe infiltrate; (H) left upper lobe;
(I) left upper lobe lateral view.
Source: Courtesy of Dr. David Begleiter.

is identified and clinically correlated, a diagnosis of pneumonia or pneumonitis is given. The patient then must have repeat films in 3 to 4 weeks demonstrating resolution. If there is little to no change or an increase in the identified opacity, then a CT scan may be ordered to further investigate the identified area, which may be representative of a mass or tumor.

When evaluating consolidation, one wants to note if the heart borders or diaphragm are obscured or are shadowed by the area of consolidation. If the consolidation is located posterior to the heart, then the edges will not be obliterated. However, if the area of consolidation is anterior, it will obscure the borders.

PNEUMOTHORAX

Pneumothorax occurs when air inside the thoracic cavity becomes trapped outside the lung in the pleural space. Since the lung is a negative pressure system, any interruption within or outside of the system can cause a pneumothorax to occur. The mechanism of a pneumothorax results when inspired air escapes to an area outside the lung but within the chest cavity. This trapped air increases with each inspiration, resulting in increased intra-thoracic pressure within the affected side; thus, causing the lung to collapse. The air can even migrate to the subcutaneous tissues resulting in subcutaneous emphysema.

A pneumothorax may be spontaneous, caused by blunt or penetrating trauma, or occur secondary to an invasive procedure such as surgery or central line placement. A pneumothorax can also be caused secondary to asthma or chronic obstructive pulmonary disease (COPD), bleb rupture, pulmonary infections, neoplasm, Marfan syndrome, or smoking cocaine. Findings on a radiograph indicative of a pneumothorax are absence of lung markings throughout the birdcage **(Figure 5.6)**. This may be more apparent in the apices of the lung or top of the birdcage. A small pneumothorax may be identified by noting a darker shade of gray or black in the apex of one lung, which is representative of the air that is being trapped and pushing or replacing that segment of lung tissue. Identification of a pneumothorax is best demonstrated on an expiration view. Subcutaneous emphysema appears as intermittent areas of radiolucency and gives the soft tissues a fluffy appearance. The "ginko leaf sign"—striations of gas along the pectoralis major—has been described.

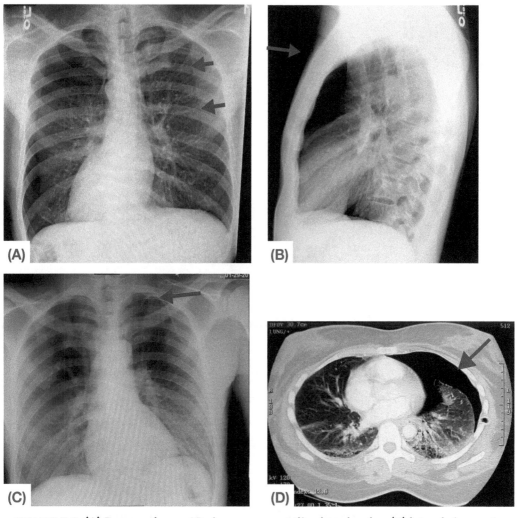

FIGURE 5.6 (A) Pneumothorax AP view: arrows outline lung border; (B) lateral view: note the free air behind the sternum; (C) after pigtail insertion; (D) CT scan demonstrating a left-sided pneumothorax.

Source: (A–C) Courtesy of Theresa M Campo; (D) courtesy of Clinical Cases (https://en.wikipedia.org/wiki/File:Pneumothorax_CT.jpg).

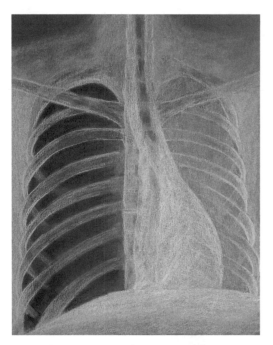

FIGURE 5.7 Tension pneumothorax.
Source: Drawing by Jody Glenn.

TENSION PNEUMOTHORAX

If a pneumothorax extends or is left untreated, it can cause a tension pneumothorax. A tension pneumothorax results in a shifting of the trachea and mediastinum away from the collapse due to the high cavity pressure. This can be identified on a plain radiograph easily **(Figure 5.7)**.

PNEUMOMEDIASTINUM

Pneumomediastinum is free air that can be found within the mediastinum as well as the soft tissue of the chest cavity, chest wall, or neck **(Figure 5.8)**. It can result from asthma, surgery, a traumatic tracheobronchial rupture, increased intrathoracic pressure, ruptured esophagus, barotrauma, or smoking crack cocaine. On plain radiographs, streaky lucencies over the mediastinum may extend up into the neck or cause elevation of the

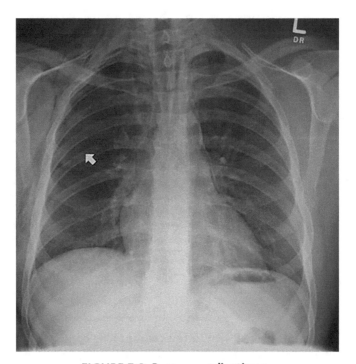

FIGURE 5.8 Pneumomediastinum.
Source: Reprinted by permission of James Heilman, MD, Wikipedian, ER Department Head, East Kootenay Regional Hospital, Clinical Assistant Professor, Department of Emergency Medicine, University of British Columbia.

parietal pleura along the mediastinal borders. When looking at a chest x-ray it is important to evaluate the entire image of the pleural cavity, including the neck and soft tissues, to identify possible free air.

HYPERAERATION

Hyperaeration may be caused by asthma or COPD, producing both subtle and overt findings on plain radiographs. Emphysema causes a loss of normal elastic recoil of the lung and destruction of the pulmonary capillary bed and alveolar septa. Diffuse hyperinflation of the lungs can cause flattening of both diaphragms, increasing the retrosternal space. Radiographic findings include prominent central pulmonary artery vasculature with rapid tapering from decreased markings, giving a pruned appearance, hyperlucency due to increased aeration and lung volume, depression or "flattening" of the diaphragmatic curves, and blunting of the costophrenic angles (Figure 5.9).

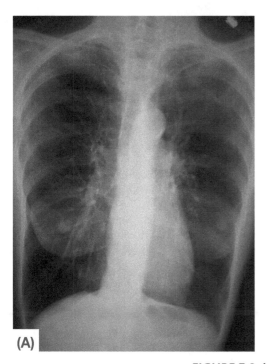
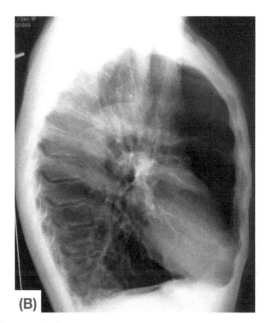

(A)   **(B)**

FIGURE 5.9 Hyperaeration.
Source: Reprinted by permission of James Heilman, MD, Wikipedian, ER Department Head, East Kootenay Regional Hospital, Clinical Assistant Professor, Department of Emergency Medicine, University of British Columbia.

MASSES AND TUMORS

Masses, or pulmonary nodules, of the lung and mediastinum are common and can be identified on plain radiographs. They may appear as single or multiple densities. If visualized, it is important to compare the image with any prior chest radiographs to determine if the finding is new or has changed or increased over time.

There are different types of masses that may be seen on a plain film including cancer, abscesses, hematomas, cysts, lymphadenopathy, and changes suggestive of lymphoma or tuberculosis (Figure 5.10). The diagnostic impression requires a thorough history and

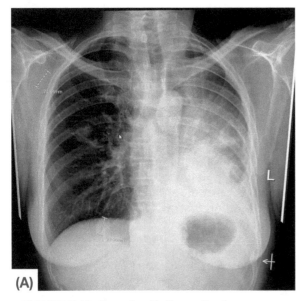 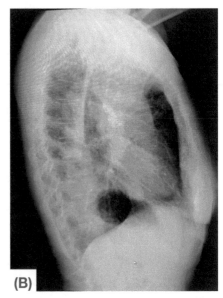

FIGURE 5.10 Complex findings of pulmonary masses involving the right lung: (A) AP view and (B) lateral view. Note the left pleural fluid, lobar collapse, and tumor.
Source: Courtesy of Theresa M. Campo.

physical examination and may require further testing to definitively identify the mass and its etiology.

It may be difficult to identify the exact location of a mass because the mediastinum is arbitrarily divided into areas of overlapping structures and compartments. Generally, masses in the mediastinum appear more clearly than masses that originate in the lung and often compress or displace other structures within the mediastinum. Masses originating in the lungs are usually surrounded by lung tissue and are less distinct. Once a mass is suspected, further diagnostic testing with CT scan or MRI may be needed to confirm the exact type of lesion. Understanding how to differentiate types of masses is beyond the intent of this text.

SARS-COV-2 (COVID-19)

The primary findings of COVID-19 on medical imaging show an atypical or organizing pneumonia. In cases that are early and mild, chest x-ray and CT scan may demonstrate normal findings in approximately 18% of patients. Findings of bilateral with or without multilobar involvement are common with distribution in the lower zones. The use of CT scan for screening is discouraged and not indicated in mild cases. Radiographs, CT scan, and ultrasonography can all be utilized for patients with COVID-19.

Common findings on radiographs are patchy, diffuse airspace opacities with either consolidation or ground glass opacity patterns **(Figure 5.11)**.

Ground glass opacities can also be seen on CT scan as well as a crazy paving pattern appearance, air space consolidation, bronchovascular thickening, tracheal bronchiectasis, and/or subpleural sparing **(Figure 5.11B–E)**.

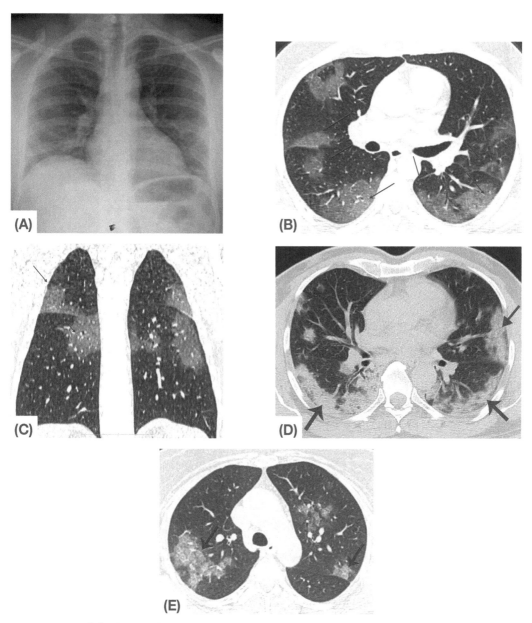

FIGURE 5.11 (A) Chest radiograph PA view demonstrates bilateral lower lobe and peripheral hazy opacities with same distribution expected to be seen on Chest CTs; (B) axial chest CT demonstrates patchy ground glass opacities with peripheral distribution; (C) coronal reconstruction chest CT of the same patient, showing patchy ground-glass opacities; (D) axial CT shows bilateral patchy consolidations, some with peripheral ground glass opacity. Findings are in peripheral and subpleural distribution. (E) COVID-19 axial chest CT shows bilateral patchy ground glass opacities with septal thickening (crazy-paving).

Source: Reproduced with permission from Chalian, H. (2022). *Coronavirus disease 2019 (COVID-19) radiologic images*. https://emedicine.medscape.com/article/2500131-overview.

CONCLUSION

The ability to identify normal and abnormal findings on a chest radiograph will become easier once you begin looking at them yourself. Comparing one's interpretation with a radiologist's final reading is an excellent way to improve your skills. If there is something identified or not identified by the radiologist, examine the films again. You may be able to visualize the area noted in the report, which will help you identify subtle findings on other images. Establishing a working relationship with radiology colleagues will also enhance your knowledge and proficiency.

RESOURCES

Au-Yong, I., Au-Yong, A., & Broderick, N. (2010). On-call x-rays made easy. Churchill Livingstone, Elsevier.

Bell, D. J. (2022). *Covid-19.* https://radiopaedia.org/articles/covid-19-4?lang=us

Chalian, H. (2022). *Coronavirus disease 2019 (COVID-19) radiologic images.* https://emedicine.medscape.com/article/2500131-overview

Collins, J., & Stern, E. J. (2008). Chest radiology: The essentials (2nd ed.). Wolters Kluwer/Lippincott Williams & Wilkins.

Goodman, L. R. (2015). Felson's principles of chest roentgenology: A programmed text (4th ed.). Elsevier Saunders.

Green, C. E., & Klein, J. S. (2012). Pulmonary vascular disease. In W. E. Brant & C. A. Helms (Eds.), Fundamentals of diagnostic radiology (4th ed., pp. 396–409). Wolters Kluwer/Lippincott Williams & Wilkins.

Herring, W. (2016). Learning radiology: Recognizing the basics (3rd ed., pp. 35–84, 97–113). Elsevier.

Klein, J. S. (2012). Airway disease. In W. E. Brant & C. A. Helms (Eds.), Fundamentals of diagnostic radiology (4th ed., pp. 487–503). Wolters Kluwer/Lippincott Williams & Wilkins.

Klein, J. S. (2012). Pulmonary infection. In W. E. Brant & C. A. Helms (Eds.), Fundamentals of diagnostic radiology (4th ed., pp. 435–452). Wolters Kluwer/Lippincott Williams & Wilkins.

Klein, J. S. (2012). Pulmonary neoplasm. In W. E. Brant & C. A. Helms (Eds.), Fundamentals of diagnostic radiology (4th ed., pp. 410–434). Wolters Kluwer/Lippincott Williams & Wilkins.

Klein, J. S., & Ghostine, J. S. (2012). Pulmonary vascular disease. In W. E. Brant & C. A. Helms (Eds.), Fundamentals of diagnostic radiology (4th ed., pp. 504–535). Wolters Kluwer/Lippincott Williams & Wilkins.

Klein, J. S., & Green, C. E. (2012). Diffuse lung disease. In W. E. Brant & C. A. Helms (Eds.), Fundamentals of diagnostic radiology (4th ed., pp. 453–486). Wolters Kluwer/Lippincott Williams & Wilkins.

Mueller, J. S., & Daffner, R. H. (2014). Chest imaging. In R. H. Daffner & M. S. Hartman (Eds.), Clinical radiology: The essentials (4th ed., pp. 79–162). Wolters Kluwer/Lippincott Williams & Wilkins.

Sciacca, F. (2021). *Covid-19 summary.* https://radiopaedia.org/articles/covid-19-summary?lang=us

CHAPTER 6

Basic Interpretation of Radiographs of the Abdomen

▶ **VIDEOS**

6.1: Interpretation of the Abdomen—Normal
6.2: Interpretation of the Abdomen—Free Air
6.3: Interpretation of the Abdomen—Small and Large Bowel Abnormalities

Accompanying videos can be accessed online at https://connect.springerpub
.com/content/book/978-0-8261-6047-8/chapter/ch06

Abdominal radiographs can be beneficial in evaluating for intestinal perforation and small and large bowel obstruction, as well as for identifying foreign bodies, renal calculi, and gallstones. Traditionally, radiographs were used in diagnosing these disorders; however, with the advent and progression of technology, other studies may be utilized, such as ultrasound, CT scan, or MRI. The benefit to abdominal radiographs is that they are inexpensive and easily obtained.

An adequate, well-penetrated, erect abdominal x-ray, as well as the use of the left decubitus view (if the patient is unable to sit or stand), can identify as little as 1 mL of free air. To evaluate an obstruction, the erect chest x-ray and supine abdominal view are not only beneficial in identifying an obstruction but also reveal infiltrates or consolidation in the lower lobes of the lungs, which may be the source of abdominal pain. The supine view is also beneficial in identifying renal calculi. However, some facilities are replacing the use of plain films with CT scan without contrast to not only rule out stones but also to evaluate for hydronephrosis.

Plain abdominal films can identify the presence of renal and ureteral calculi, and monitor their progress, utilizing far less radiation than a CT scan. Additionally, they are less expensive for the patient than a CT scan. An obstruction series can be beneficial in identifying radiopaque foreign bodies that are either ingested or placed in the anus or vagina. It can also be used to track the progression, or lack thereof, of an already established ureteral stone. CT has become exclusively used in many facilities even though plain radiographs are not only important, but are cost-effective. It is important to have a firm foundation and knowledge of anatomy, physiology, and pathophysiology when reviewing any radiographic study.

INTERPRETATION AND NORMAL FINDINGS

To begin the interpretation of abdominal films, one must utilize the ABCDEFs. The ABCDEFs for abdominal films are slightly different from those used when evaluating chest films. The ABCs allow you to identify normal from abnormal with an organized consistent approach. The ABCs are:

Adequacy/**A**ir—free intraperitoneal air rises to the anterior region (front) of the abdomen when the patient is supine, so it is best viewed on erect films if a perforation is suspected **(Figure 6.1)**. Remember, hot air rises and can identify the presence of intraperitoneal air as well as intestinal air–fluid levels **(Figure 6.2)**. Visualize the small and large intestines and assess air–fluid levels and caliber of the intestinal lumen.

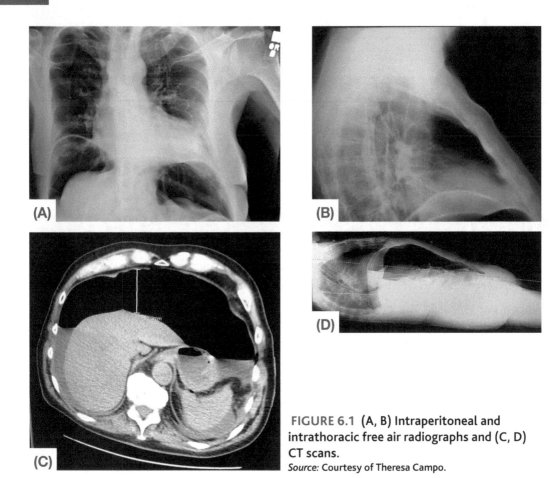

FIGURE 6.1 (A, B) Intraperitoneal and intrathoracic free air radiographs and (C, D) CT scans.
Source: Courtesy of Theresa Campo.

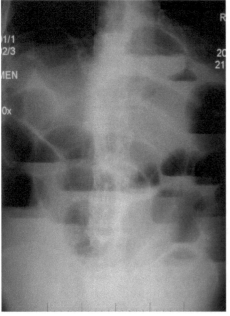

FIGURE 6.2 Intestinal air–fluid levels.
Source: Courtesy of Dr. David Begleiter.

*B*owel gas patterns—the small bowel lies in the center of the abdomen. It is of smaller caliber, approximately 3 cm, than the colon and contains air and fluid. The large bowel lies peripherally and contains feces, especially in the distal aspects, and there is no definite measurement as it varies based on the stool content; however, it should not measure more than 5.5 cm. Haustra are present in the large bowel but not in small bowel, allowing one to differentiate the two. Gas and air rise anteriorly while in the supine position and are best viewed in the erect view, demonstrating air in the stomach, transverse colon, and sigmoid colon **(Figure 6.3)**.

Calcification—calcifications can be seen and may be normal or abnormal. Phleboliths, which are small calcified veins in the pelvis, are often confused with stones in the urinary tract. More than 90% of renal stones can be visualized on a plain film. In 10% to 15% of patients, gallstones can also be visualized on a plain film **(Figure 6.4)**.

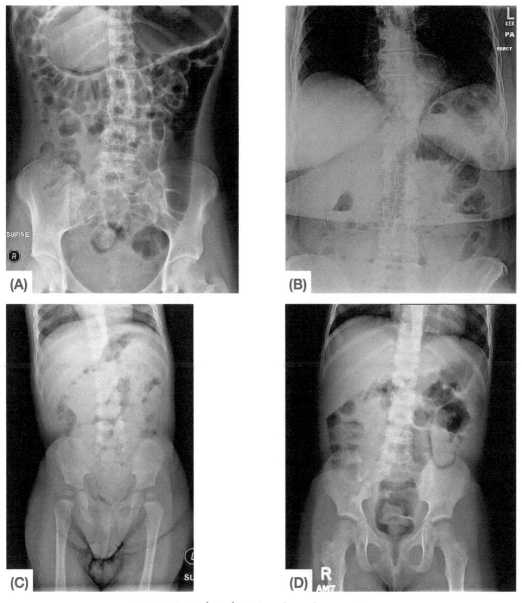

FIGURE 6.3 (A–D) Various bowel gas patterns.
Source: Courtesy of Dr. David Begleiter.

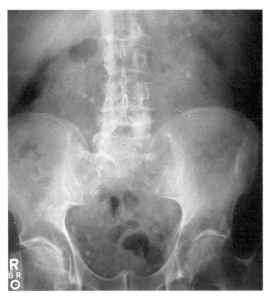

FIGURE 6.4 Calcifications/stones. Note the various densities above the pelvis and within the main ring of the pelvis.
Source: Courtesy of Bill Rhodes/Wikipedia Commons.

Densities—radiopaque foreign bodies, whether ingested or inserted, can be identified on plain radiographs as radiographic densities **(Figure 6.5)**.

Edges—The bowel and gastric folds can be identified and aid in identifying abnormal findings. The bowel wall should not be more than 3 mm thick. The small and large bowel should not be more than 3 cm in diameter and the cecum should never exceed 9 cm in diameter. Gastric folds should be parallel to the long axis of the stomach and the small bowel folds should be followed from one side to the other. In the large bowel, the haustral folds do not go from side to side but go partially across on each side—they do not meet **(Figure 6.6)**.

Fat plane—fat plane may be normally visualized on the abdominal radiographs but often represent an abnormality. If a fat plane is identified in the psoas, perirenal, perivesical, or retroperitoneal areas, this is abnormal and must be further evaluated with other diagnostic studies **(Figure 6.7)**.

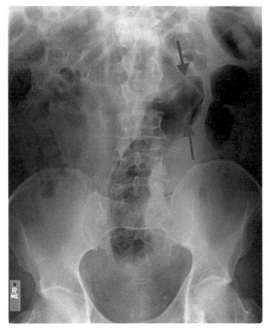

FIGURE 6.5 Foreign body.
Source: Pandey, B. B., Dang, T. C., & Healy, J. F. (2005). Embolic stroke complicating *Staphylococcus aureus* endocarditis circumstantially linked to rectal trauma from foreign body: A first case report. *BMC Infectious Diseases, 5*, 42. https://doi.org/10.1186/1471-2334-5-42. https://commons.wikimedia.org/wiki/File:Rectal_foreign_body_04.jpg

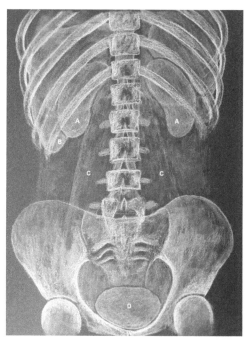

FIGURE 6.6 Edges (A, kidney; B, lung; C, psoas muscle; D, bladder).
Source: Drawing by Jodi Glenn.

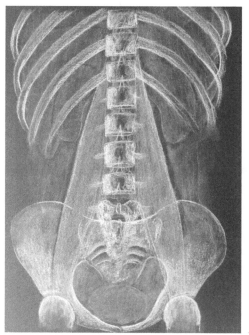

FIGURE 6.7 Fat planes.
Source: Drawing by Jodi Glenn.

Skeleton, solid organs—it is important to evaluate the skeleton throughout the abdominal series to identify any occult or obvious fractures **(Figure 6.8)**. Depending on the location and extent of the fracture, underlying organ damage must be considered. If fractures of varying age are identified, abuse must be given consideration.

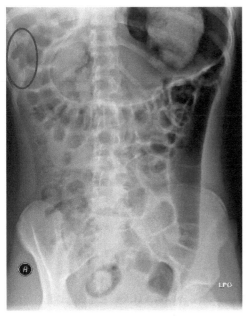

FIGURE 6.8 Skeletal fracture on abdominal film.
Source: Theresa M. Campo.

FREE AIR AND AIR–FLUID LEVELS

Intraluminal gas patterns and free air can be indicative of bowel obstruction or pneumoperitoneum. Intraluminal gas patterns can either be balanced and occur at the same level or at different levels (stair-step; **Figure 6.9**). Abnormally produced intraluminal air–fluid levels in more than one bowel loop, distention, and the presence of mucosal wall thickening are indicative of an obstruction. In the colon, air mixed with bowel contents can give a bubbly appearance and may be normal in adults, but is never normal in children and infants. Gaseous distention of the small or large bowel with air–fluid levels may be indicative of an ileus. When obstruction occurs, the bowel loops proximal to the obstruction, becomes distended/dilated, and there is paucity of gas distal to the obstruction. Distention can be significant. In the pediatric patient, intussusception can give a mass effect, target appearance (telescoping of bowel), and crescent streaking of air that outlines the trapped bowel **(Figure 6.10)**.

Extraluminal gas or free air can be indicative of pneumoperitoneum and is best visualized on an erect film **(Figure 6.11)**. If the patient is unable to sit or stand, then a lateral decubitus view can be obtained to identify the free air. Extraluminal air can be present in an abscess, retroperitoneal space, or bowel wall under the diaphragm or biliary or portal venous system of the liver. Perforation of viscous can be either intraperitoneal or retroperitoneal. The most common cause of pneumoperitoneum is either a perforated peptic ulcer or colonic diverticulum.

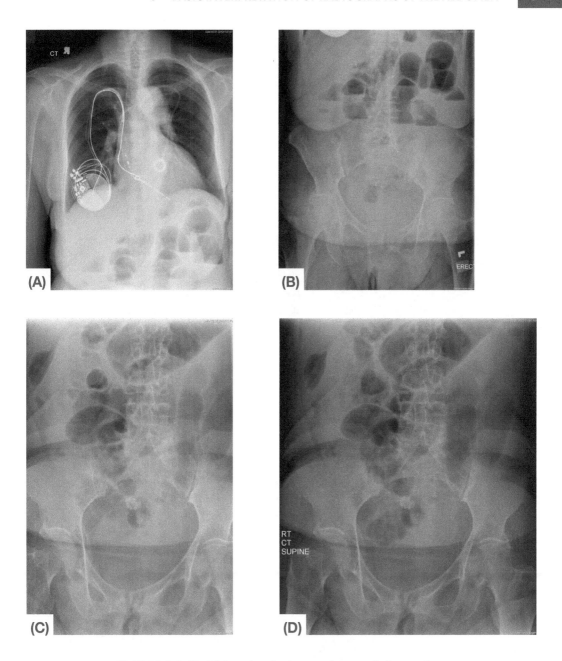

FIGURE 6.9 (A–D) Intraluminal gas patterns of obstruction.
Note the air/fluid levels and paucity of markings distal to the obstruction.
Source: Courtesy of Dr. Douglas W. Parrillo.

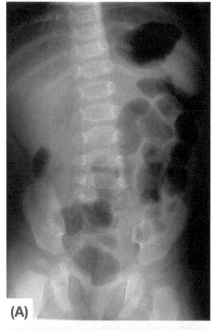

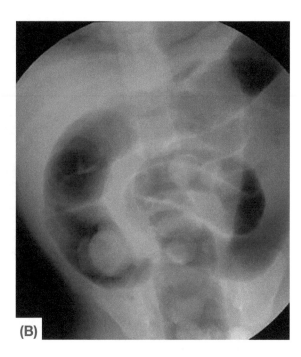

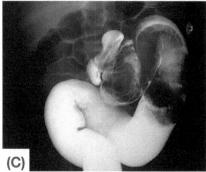

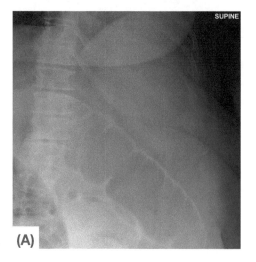

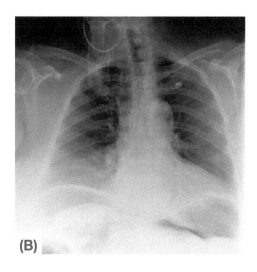

FIGURE 6.10 (A–C) Intussusception.
Source: Images reprinted with permission from Medscape Drugs &
Diseases. (2016). http://emedicine.medscape.com/article/930708
-overview

FIGURE 6.11 (A–C) Pneumoperitoneum.

(continued)

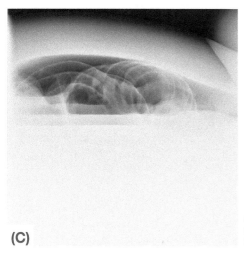

FIGURE 6.11 (*continued*)
Source: Copyright 2016 Dr. Alexandra Stanislavsky. Image courtesy of Dr. Alexandra Stanislavsky and Radiopaedia.org. Used under license.

(C)

CALCIFICATIONS

Calculi are readily visualized on abdominal films because the majority are made up of calcium or cholesterol, which can be easily visualized on radiographs. Calcifications, representing renal calculi, may be identified along the urinary tract from the kidneys down to the urethra. Gallstones can be seen within the gallbladder, and calcifications within vessels are known as fecoliths (see **Figure 6.4**).

FOREIGN BODIES

Foreign bodies in the gastrointestinal tract and genitourinary tract may be ingested or inserted. Plain radiographs of the abdomen are beneficial only if the foreign body is radiopaque and has either a high-density such as iron tablets or a metallic component within it. The object will appear as bright white on the film if it contains metal and, depending on its location, may look out of place when considering the mode in which it arrived in the area (see **Figure 6.5**).

DILATED SMALL BOWEL

The most common cause of dilated small bowel is mechanical obstruction and paralytic ileus. Mechanical obstruction may be caused by adhesions, strangulated hernia, mass, gallstones, Crohn's disease-related strictures, appendiceal abscess, volvulus, or intussusception. When evaluating the abdominal plain radiograph, the normal caliber of the small intestine should not be greater than 3 cm. If the small bowel is dilated greater than 3 cm and contains variable air and fluid levels and the large bowel is not dilated or not able to be visualized, then an obstruction must be suspected. The small bowel will have the appearance of a "string of beads" when air gets trapped between the valvulae conniventes (**Figure 6.12**). If a small bowel obstruction is suspected, then a CT scan should be considered for further investigation into the cause and extent of the obstruction.

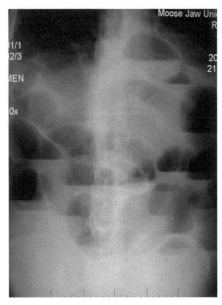

FIGURE 6.12 **Small bowel obstruction.**
Source: Reprinted by permission of James Heilman, MD, Wikipedian, ER Department Head, East Kootenay Regional Hospital, Clinical Assistant Professor, Department of Emergency Medicine, University of British Columbia.

DILATED LARGE BOWEL AND MEGACOLON

The large bowel may be visualized on the abdominal film. When large bowel dilatation is present, the colonic diameter is greater in caliber, measuring 5.5 cm, and is considered abnormal (**Figure 6.13**). Large bowel dilatation may occur with or without an obstruction and may be caused by tumors, volvulus, inflammatory bowel disease, diverticulitis, or other forms of colitis. Volvulus most often occurs in the cecum and sigmoid colon. The bird-beak sign demonstrates a sigmoid volvulus with the narrowing of the segment of colon. Perforation of the colon must be considered in patients with volvulus when the caliber of the lumen exceeds 9 cm. When large bowel dilatation occurs in patients with inflammatory bowel disease, characterized by wall thickening with mucosal edema, toxic megacolon must be considered. Thumb printing can be seen on obstruction series, suggesting possible microscopic or overt perforation (**Figure 6.14**). If a large bowel obstruction is suspected, then a CT scan should be considered for further

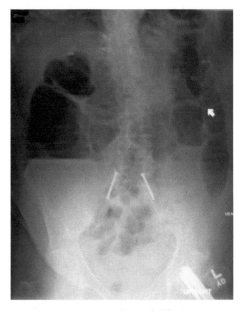

FIGURE 6.13 **Large bowel dilation.**
Source: Reprinted by permission of James Heilman, MD, Wikipedian, ER Department Head, East Kootenay Regional Hospital, Clinical Assistant Professor, Department of Emergency Medicine, University of British Columbia.

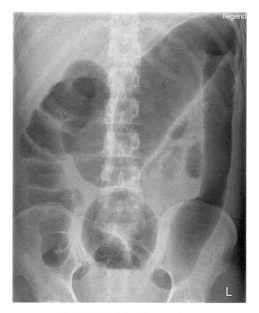

FIGURE 6.14 Megacolon.
Source: Hellerhoff. (2012). https://commons
.wikimedia.org/wiki/File:Toxisches_Megacolon_bei_Colitis_ulcerosa.jpg

evaluation. Contrasted radiographs should not be considered or used with large bowel obstruction. The barium sulfate does not dilute and can worsen an obstruction and obscure visualization with CT scan for further evaluation.

CONCLUSION

Plain abdominal radiographs can be beneficial in identifying numerous abnormalities such as free air and fluid, obstruction, perforation, foreign bodies, and calcifications within the abdominal cavity. Plain films of the abdomen are also beneficial because they are less expensive than other radiographic studies such as CT scans and MRIs. However, with the progression of technology, other more expensive testing modalities may be adopted as first-line approaches. If the patient is a female of childbearing age or a pediatric patient, ultrasound may be a beneficial alternative to abdominal radiography.

RESOURCES

Au-Yong, I., Au-Yong, A., & Broderick, N. (2010). *On-call x-rays made easy.* Churchill Livingstone, Elsevier.

Brant, W. E. (2018). Mesenteric small bowel. In. W. E. Brant & C. A. Helms (Eds.), *Fundamentals of diagnostic radiology* (5th ed., pp. 765–779). Wolters Kluwer/Lippincott Williams & Wilkins.

Brant, W. E. (2018). Stomach and duodenum. In W. E. Brant & C. A. Helms (Eds.), *Fundamentals of diagnostic radiology* (5th ed., pp. 752–764). Wolters Kluwer/Lippincott Williams & Wilkins.

Brant, W. E., & Erickson, S. (2018). Colon and appendix. In W. E. Brant & C. A. Helms (Eds.), *Fundamentals of diagnostic radiology* (5th ed., pp. 780–795). Wolters Kluwer/Lippincott Williams & Wilkins.

Brant, W. E., & Pohl, J. (2018a). Abdomen and pelvis. In W. E. Brant & C. A. Helms (Eds.), *Fundamentals of diagnostic radiology* (5th ed., pp. 670–691). Wolters Kluwer/Lippincott Williams & Wilkins.

Brant, W. E., & Pohl, J. (2018b). Liver, biliary tree and gallbladder. In W. E. Brant & C. A. Helms (Eds.), *Fundamentals of diagnostic radiology* (5th ed., pp. 692–719). Wolters Kluwer/Lippincott Williams & Wilkins.

Gay, S. B., Lambert, D. L., & Reynolds, R. (n.d.). *Introduction to abdominal plain radiographs.* https://introductiontoradiology.net/courses/rad/PlainAbdomen/

Hartman, M. S., & Daffner, R. H. (2014). Abdominal radiographs. In R. H. Daffner & M. S. Hartman (Eds.), *Clinical radiology: The essentials* (4th ed., pp. 215–251). Wolters Kluwer/Lippincott Williams & Wilkins.

Herring, W. (2016). *Learning radiology: Recognizing the basics* (3rd ed., pp. 129–139, 183–192). Elsevier.

Moshiri, S., & Brant, W. E. (2012). Pharynx and esophagus. In W. E. Brant & C. A. Helms (Eds.), *Fundamentals of diagnostic radiology* (4th ed., pp. 734–751). Wolters Kluwer/Lippincott Williams & Wilkins.

Pandey, B. B., Dang, T. C., & Healy, J. F. (2005). Embolic stroke complicating *Staphylococcus aureus* endocarditis circumstantially linked to rectal trauma from foreign body: A first case report. *BMC Infectious Diseases, 5,* 42. https://doi.org/10.1186/1471-2334-5-42. https://commons.wikimedia.org/wiki/File:Rectal_foreign_body_04.jpg

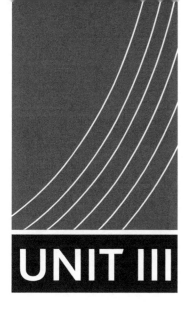

UNIT III

Interpretation of Extremity Radiographs

CHAPTER 7

Basic Interpretation of Long Bone—Upper Extremity Radiographs

Radiographs of long bones, whether of the upper extremity or the lower extremity, are usually performed after a traumatic injury. However, pain, swelling, and/or redness may also be an indication for obtaining radiographs to rule out an abnormal growth, bursitis, neoplasms, and foreign bodies. Plain radiographs of long bones are beneficial in identifying fractures, subluxation, dislocation, and soft tissue swelling in traumatic injuries and are also useful in evaluating nontraumatic signs and symptoms such as abnormal bone growths.

In this chapter, normal findings on plain radiographs are discussed along with joint structures and normal variants, as well as common findings in adults and children. Knowledge of normal anatomical structures is imperative in interpreting long-bone radiographs.

NORMAL

Before ordering a plain radiograph of a long bone or joint, it is important to review some of the rules discussed in earlier chapters. Additionally, when evaluating the upper extremity, it is important to not only evaluate the affected area, but also the joints above and below. For instance, if the patient complains of an injury to the forearm, medical imaging should include the elbow as well as the wrist. Routine studies should include a minimum of two views; most have three views or more, depending on the area in question.

Plain radiographs are excellent in identifying bony abnormalities such as fractures. Although not the best modality for evaluating soft tissue conditions surrounding a particular joint—such as cartilage, muscle, and tendons, which are best seen using MRI—plain films do show changes within joint alignment and edema, which are indicative of an occult bone fracture, trauma, or inflammation. An example of an occult fracture finding is when the posterior fat pad, which is only visible if bleeding occurs within the joint space, is viewed on the lateral view of an elbow and the anterior fat pad appears like the sail of a sailboat, which is suggestive of a radial head fracture that may not be seen in the bony cortex (**Figure 7.1**).

The upper extremity consists of the shoulder, elbow, wrist, and phalangeal joints and associated bones: humerus, radius, ulna, carpal, metacarpal, and phalanges. Each joint and each bone have different appearances as well as functions within the upper extremity. Abnormalities can cause inhibition of normal function and use of the upper extremity. There are five types of bones in the body, as shown in **Table 7.1**. When evaluating bones on a radiograph, scan the cortical margins and note alignment to identify an abnormality.

The ABCs of interpretation can be utilized for systematic assessment of the upper extremity. *A* is for **a**dequacy and **a**lignment. As stated in previous chapters, adequacy of the film is of the utmost importance when evaluating any radiographs. Proper alignment allows the viewer to identify subtle joint abnormalities. It does not only refer to the alignment of one particular bone, but also alignment within the joint (**Figure 7.2A**). *B* is for **b**ones and refers to the evaluation of all components of the bone in the respective study. Cortical margins and borders should be evaluated for any disruption or lack of continuity of that

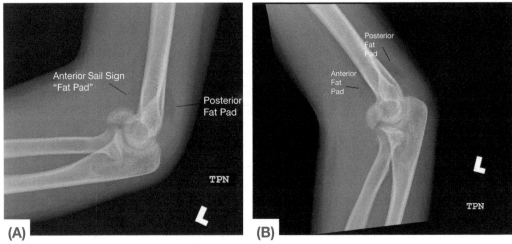

FIGURE 7.1 **(A) Anterior and posterior and (B) lateral fat pad sign in the elbow.**
Source: Courtesy of Dr. Douglas W. Parrillo; diagramming by Theresa M. Campo.

TABLE 7.1 FIVE TYPES OF BONES WITH DEFINITION AND EXAMPLES

TYPE OF BONE	DEFINITION	EXAMPLE
Long bone	The length is greater than the width	Femur, humerus, phalanges
Short bone	The length and width are comparable	Cuboid bones, carpals, tarsals
Flat bone	Diploic bones	Skull
Sesmoid bone	Small round bones that are located in tendons	Foot and hand
Irregular bone	Irregularly shaped	Vertebrae, sacrum

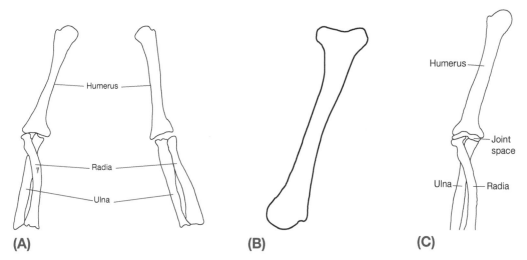

FIGURE 7.2 (A) Alignment of upper extremity bones; (B) intact bony cortex;
(C) joint space.
Source: Drawing courtesy of Theresa M. Campo.

bone indicative of a fracture. It also refers to any abnormal growths or appearances, which may appear as densities or opacities on the radiographic image **(Figure 7.2B)**. Cartilage and joints can be evaluated for abnormalities with visualization of the joint space. Loss of any joint space may be indicative of a crush injury or could be a sign of degenerative joint disease. Bulging or displacement of normal structures in the lower extremity may be indicative of a joint effusion **(Figure 7.2C)**. Soft tissue can give signs of trauma with the joint effusion or edema. It can also assist the provider in identifying radiopaque foreign bodies that may have occurred during the injury itself.

ABNORMALITIES OF THE UPPER EXTREMITY

Fractures

DESCRIBING FRACTURES

A fracture or break to a bone or bones can happen from injury or pathology. Simply describing a fracture is important when documenting findings, but it is also important to utilize the proper terminology when describing these findings. A fracture line or pattern may be transverse, oblique, spiral, comminuted, impacted, avulsed, compressed, or depressed. A fracture may only involve one side of the bone, may involve both sides, or may go completely through the bone itself **(Figure 7.3)**. A normal variant that may be visualized involves blood vessels along the bone appearing as fractures. These can be differentiated from a fracture by tracing the lines and seeing if they pass the normal border of the bone (cortex). However, it is important to note that both may go through the cortex; many vascular channels traverse the cortex and make differentiating difficult.

Fractures may involve one bone or multiple bones. There may also be multiple fractures within the same bone but in different areas. The bone fragments may be displaced or nondisplaced. When a bone fragment is 100% displaced, causing shortening and overlapping of the bone fragments, this is known as a bayonet deformity **(Figure 7.4)**. When the

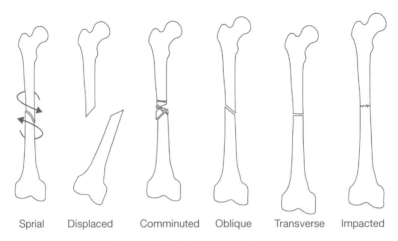

Sprial Displaced Comminuted Oblique Transverse Impacted

FIGURE 7.3 Fracture patterns.
Source: Drawing by Ocean City High School student.

bone fragments are out of alignment with each other, they are considered to be angulated. Angulation is the angle between the longitudinal axis of the main fracture fragment and the other fragment. Significant angulation requires reduction and realignment of the bone fragments. If the fracture line is forced into the joint space, it is considered to be an intraarticular fracture **(Figure 7.5)**.

A stress fracture can occur with repetitious loading beyond the bone tolerance. An avulsion fracture may occur when there is a forcible muscular contraction of tendinous (tendon attaches muscle to bone, whereas ligament attaches bone to bone) attachment to a bone that is pulled off and away from the main structure.

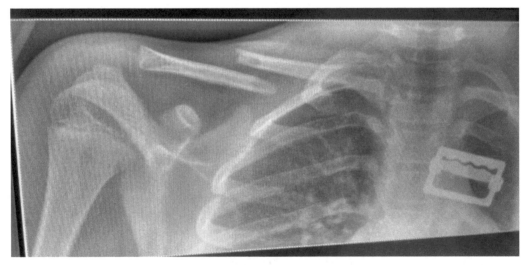

FIGURE 7.4 Bayonet deformity.
Source: Courtesy of Theresa M. Campo.

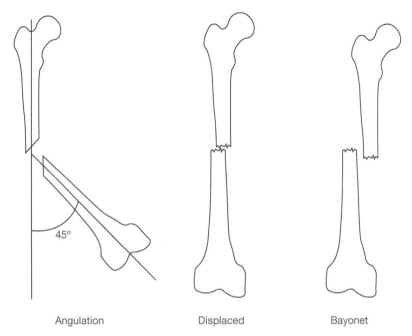

FIGURE 7.5 Angulation, displacement, and a bayonet deformity.
Source: Drawing by Ocean City High School student.

PEDIATRIC CONSIDERATIONS

Special consideration needs to be given with regard to the pediatric patient. Pediatric bones are more fibrous and less crystalline (or calcified) than adult bones. They are enclosed in a sheet of strong fibrous periosteum and have epiphyseal growth plates, which are a zone of weakness. Children tend to have incomplete fractures such as a greenstick fracture or torus fracture because the bone ends do not separate as in adults because of the strong periosteal sleeve. The most common types of fractures in the pediatric patient are elastic deformation, bowing deformation, torus or buckle fracture, greenstick fracture, Salter–Harris fracture, stress injury, and avulsion injury **(Figure 7.6)**.

Pediatric bones have epiphyseal growth plates that allow the bones to grow until they are mature adult bones. When a fracture occurs within or around the growth plate, it can complicate the healing process. Gross disturbances can be expected and the potential for loss of growth of the long bones may occur. However, current literature demonstrates that the loss of length after a fracture of a long bone tends to be made up in 1 to 2 years after the injury by overgrowth. The epiphyseal growth plate is a zone of weakness that can make fracture, separation, and slipping of the growth plate more common in the pediatric patient.

The Salter–Harris classification system is used to describe the five different types of pediatric growth plate fractures based on abnormalities involving either the metaphysis, epiphysis, and/or diaphysis. A Salter–Harris I fracture is a separation of the growth plate without involvement of the metaphysis or the epiphysis. A Salter–Harris II fracture occurs across the growth plate but with a small fragment of metaphysis remaining attached to the epiphysis. A fracture across the growth plate with extension of the fracture line across the epiphysis is known as a Salter–Harris III fracture. When the fracture line traverses the epiphysis and part of the diaphysis, this is known as a Salter–Harris IV fracture. Finally, when there is damage to both the epiphysis and the metaphysis from a crush injury, this is known as a Salter–Harris V fracture. As you will notice, the severity of the injury increases with the designating number of the Salter–Harris fracture (Figure 7.7). An easy mnemonic to remember the Salter classification is SALTR: s refers to a *slip* as in a Salter–Harris I, **a** refers to the fracture noted **a***bove* or proximal to the epiphyseal plate, **l** refers to a fracture be**l***ow* or distal to the epiphyseal plate, **t** is a fracture line extending **t***hrough* the epiphyseal plate including both the epiphysis and metaphysis, and **r** refers to c**r***ush*.

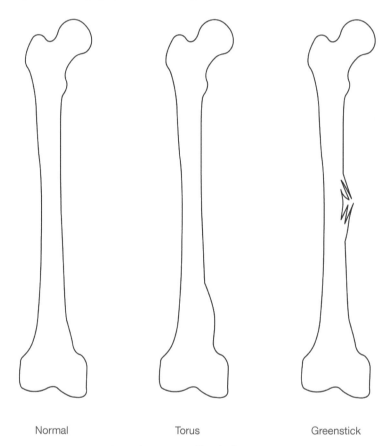

Normal   Torus   Greenstick

FIGURE 7.6 Pediatric fractures.
Source: Drawing by Ocean City High School student.

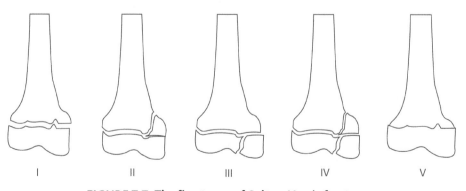

I   II   III   IV   V

FIGURE 7.7 The five types of Salter–Harris fractures.
Source: Drawing by Ocean City High School student.

Another useful mnemonic is SALTEr. The letters refer to *s*pace, *a*bove, *l*ower, *t*hrough, and *e*rase: *s*pace refers to a fracture in the space visualized on the x-ray, *a*bove and *l*ower refer to the fracture relationship to the growth plate, *t*hrough refers to the fracture passing through the growth plate and therefore appearing on both sides, and **e***rase* refers to erasing the appearance of the growth plate on the x-ray (this is synonymous with "crush" in the above example).

SHOULDER

Alignment of the glenohumeral joint should demonstrate the humeral head lying in the glenoid fossa. The distance between the humeral head in the anterior margin of the glenoid should be equal from top to bottom **(Figure 7.8)**. If the humeral head is internally rotated and looks like a light bulb on a plain radiograph, suspect a posterior dislocation. Alignment of the acromioclavicular joint should show alignment of the inferior margins of the lateral end of the clavicle and acromium.

The shoulder is made up of three bones: the clavicle, the humerus, and the scapula. The scapula provides support and stability to the shoulder through three structures where tendons and ligaments attach. The coracoid process is in the anterior plane of the shoulder blade and the acromion is in the posterior region. These structures are supported by the coracoacromial ligament. The humeral head is adjacent to the glenoid portion of the scapula and is supported by the muscles, tendons, and ligaments that make up the rotator cuff. This region is referred to as the glenohumeral joint. The distal aspect of the clavicle, adjacent to the acromium, comprises the acromioclavicular joint. A fracture of any of the bony structures within the shoulder or a soft tissue injury to the rotator cuff ligaments and/or tendons results in shoulder instability, loss of function, and pain **(Figure 7.8)**.

Shoulder injuries are common in all age groups and may consist of a fracture, dislocation, or both occurring simultaneously. Clavicular fractures are the most common fractures in children and adolescents. Shoulder dislocation and acromioclavicular (AC) separations are most common in adults. In the elderly, the most common injury is fracture of the humerus, particularly the head and neck. If soft tissue injury is suspected and a dislocation and/or fracture has been ruled in or out with plain radiographs, an MRI should be considered for better visualization of the soft tissue structures.

Radiographic studies of the shoulder should have three views: the anterior–posterior (AP) view, axial view, and the "Y" view **(Figure 7.9)**. The AP view allows for viewing the contour of each bone, which should

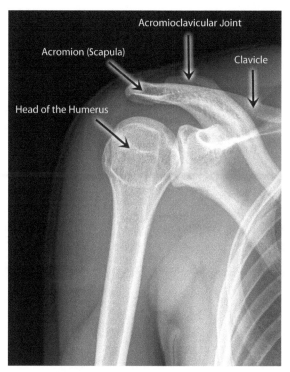

FIGURE 7.8 Shoulder anatomy.
Source: **Campo, T., & Lafferty, K. A. (2021).** *Essential procedures for emergency, urgent, and primary care settings* (**3rd ed.**). **Springer Publishing Company.**

be evaluated systematically. One should note that the cortices are smooth and visible ribs should also be evaluated. In the axial view, identification of the coracoid process should be visualized. The axial view is also useful in assessing the glenohumeral alignment for evaluation of any avulsions of the glenoid rim and for a Hill–Sachs defect of the humeral head. The "Y" view is beneficial for confirming normal alignment of the glenohumeral joint and identification of either an anterior or posterior dislocation.

As children grow and develop, so do their bones. There is formation of ossification centers of the humerus, scapula, and clavicle, which are formed over years and eventually fuse. Table 7.2 demonstrates the time of formation and time of fusion of the secondary ossification centers.

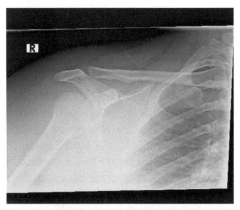
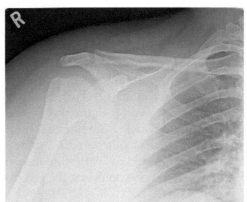
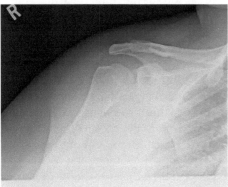

FIGURE 7.9 **Three views of a shoulder radiograph.**
Source: Courtesy of Dr. David Begleiter.

TABLE 7.2 OSSIFICATION CENTER FORMATION AND FUSION

SHOULDER BONE OSSIFICATION CENTER	FORMATION (AGE)	FUSION (AGE)
Humeral head	<6 months	16–18 years
Humerus/greater tuberosity	1 year	4–6 years
Humerus/lesser tuberosity	5 years	7 years
Scapula/coracoid	1 year	20 years
Scapula/inferior angle	15 years	15 years
Scapula/acromium	15 years	20–25 years
Clavicle/medial margin	18 years	25 years

CLAVICLE

Clavicle fractures can occur from minimal force and most often occur in the midshaft and distal aspect (Figure 7.10). Midshaft clavicle fractures may be seen more frequently in younger individuals, especially those younger than 20 or 21 years of age. Fractures of the lateral/distal aspects are more common in older individuals. The skin overlying a clavicle

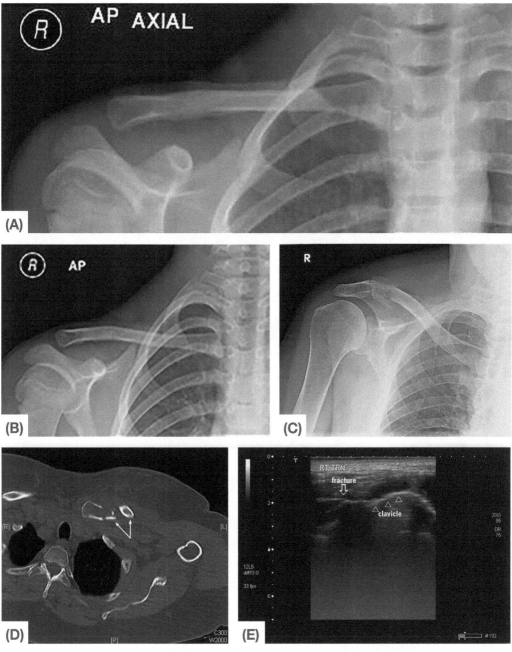

FIGURE 7.10 **(A,B)** Normal clavicle; **(C)** distal clavicle fracture; **(D)** medial clavicular fracture without injury to the sternoclavicular (SC) joint; **(E)** ultrasonogram of a clavicular fracture.
Source: (A–C) Courtesy of Dr. David Begleiter; (D,E) reproduced with permission from Medscape Drugs & Diseases. https://emedicine.medscape.com/, Imaging of Clavicular Fractures and Dislocations. (2022). https://emedicine.medscape.com/article/398799-overview

fracture should be assessed for tenting that is causing skin displacement. Tenting can result when fracture fragments protrude and pinch the skin. These fracture fragments may need to be repaired, requiring surgical intervention. One should suspect an intrathoracic injury with any proximal clavicle fracture, such as pneumothorax or pneumomediastinum.

Clavicle fractures can also be visualized using CT scan and ultrasonography. **Figure 7.10D** demonstrates a medial clavicular fracture without injury to the sternoclavicular (SC) joint and **Figure 7.10E** demonstrates an ultrasonogram of a clavicular fracture.

SCAPULA

Fractures to the scapulaa result from a great deal of direct force and have a high correlation of injury to the thorax, head, and spine. When evaluating or identifying a scapular fracture, it is imperative that the provider completely evaluate all of the surrounding structures for accompanying injury. Scapular fractures can be difficult to identify and visualize on a plain radiograph. Obtaining a "Y" view is most beneficial, but MRI or CT scanning may be necessary for a definitive diagnosis **(Figures 7.11, 7.12, and 7.13)**.

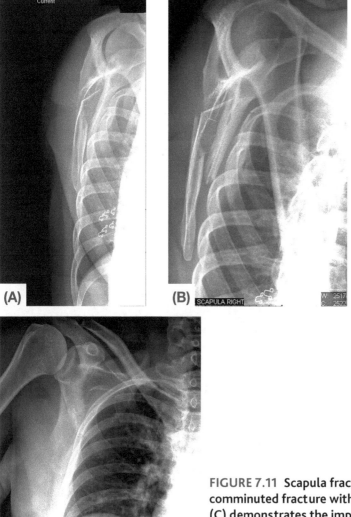

FIGURE 7.11 Scapula fractures: (A,B) Note the comminuted fracture with multiple bone fragments; (C) demonstrates the importance of more than one view for visualization of the fracture.
Source: Courtesy of Dr. David Begleiter.

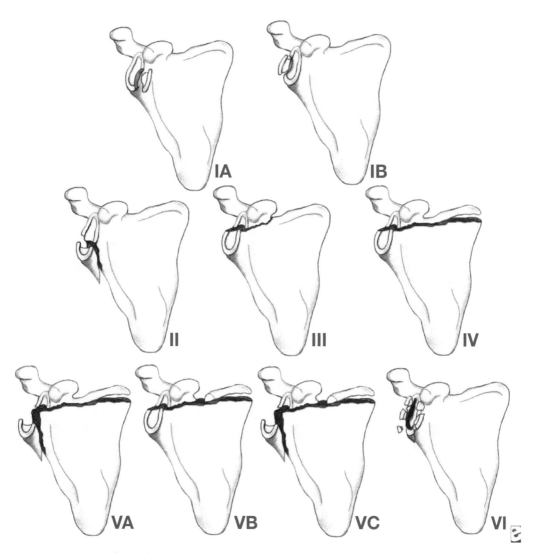

FIGURE 7.12 Glenoid cavity fractures are classified based on the location and type of fracture (i.e., displacement and combination of fractures): IA, anterior rim fracture; IB, posterior rim fracture; II, fracture line through the glenoid fossa exiting at the lateral border of the scapula; III, fracture line through the glenoid fossa exiting at the superior border of the scapula; IV, fracture line through the glenoid fossa exiting at the medial border of the scapula; VA, combination of types II and IV; VB, combination of types III and IV; VC, combination of types II, III, and IV; VI, comminuted fracture.

Source: Reproduced with permission from Medscape Drugs & Diseases. https://emedicine.medscape.com/, Scapula Fracture (2022). https://emedicine.medscape.com/article/1263076-overview

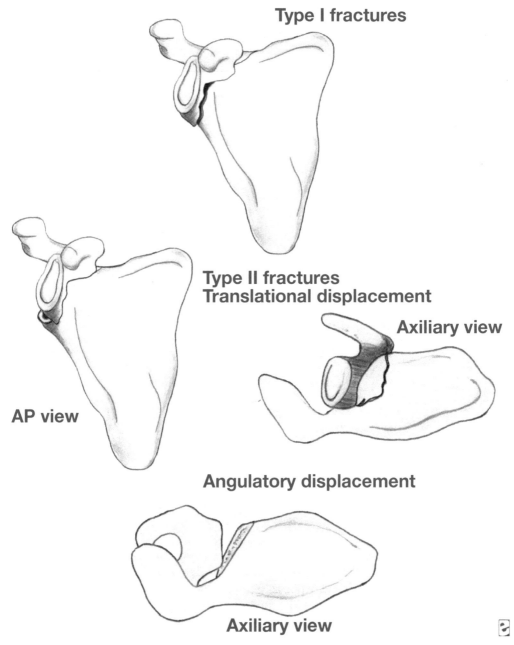

FIGURE 7.13 Glenoid neck fractures are classified based on the location and type of fracture (i.e., displacement, and combination of fractures). Type I includes all minimally displaced fractures. Type II includes all significantly displaced fractures (translational displacement greater than or equal to 1 cm; angulatory displacement greater than or equal to 40°).

Source: Reproduced with permission from Medscape Drugs & Diseases. https://emedicine.medscape.com/, Scapula Fracture (2022). https://emedicine.medscape.com/article/1263076-overview

HUMERUS

There are four parts to the proximal humerus: the greater tuberosity, lesser tuberosity, head, and neck leading to the shaft (Figure 7.14). Proximal humeral fractures have a peak incidence during adolescence, causing epiphyseal separation. Fracture of this region in adults aged 45 years and older is most often due to osteoporosis. A fall with an outstretched hand is one of the more common mechanisms for fracture of the proximal humerus. If a fracture occurs in the humeral neck, it may be accompanied by complications from neurovascular injury, avascular necrosis, and adhesive capsulitis. A compression fracture of the posterolateral humeral head is known as a Hill–Sachs fracture and may be caused by anterior glenohumeral dislocation and impaction of the humeral head against the anterior glenoid rim.

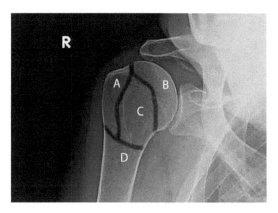

FIGURE 7.14 Four parts of the proximal humerus: (A) greater tuberosity; (B) humeral head; (C) lesser tuberosity; (D) humeral neck going into the shaft.
Courtesy of Dr. David Begleiter.

Fractures to the shaft of the humerus may be complicated by injury to the radial nerve with entrapment or impingement. When a fracture occurs in the distal third of the humerus involving radial nerve entrapment, this is known as a Holstein–Lewis fracture (Figure 7.15).

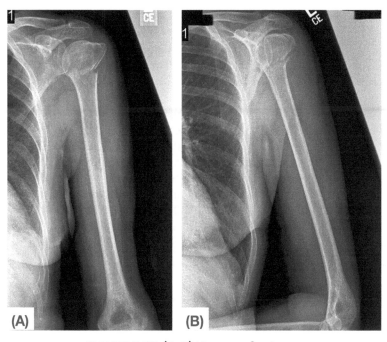

(A)   (B)

FIGURE 7.15 (A–B) Humerus fractures.

(continued)

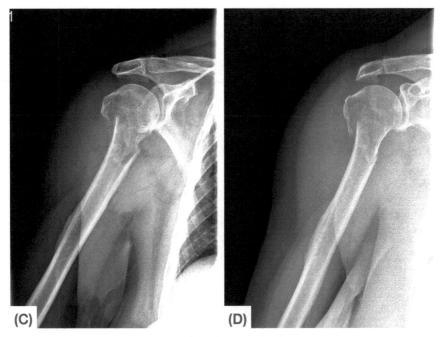

FIGURE 7.15 (C–D) Humerus fractures.
Source: Courtesy of Dr. David Begleiter and Theresa M. Campo.

ELBOW

The elbow joint consists of the distal humerus and the proximal radius and ulna. The distal humerus consists of the medial and lateral epicondyle, coronoid fossa, capitellum, and trochlea **(Figure 7.16)**. The radial head, radial tuberosity, ulnar tuberosity, and olecranon process are key areas when evaluating an elbow image. The ulna and olecranon process articulate with the trochlea and the olecranon fossa of the humerus. The radial head articulates with the capitellum allowing pronation and supination of the forearm, and the two structures should be aligned in all projections. Trauma to the elbow occurs in all ages but most commonly in children. Elbow fractures in children require emergent orthopedic consultation to avoid permanent deformity and loss of function. It is important to obtain an AP, lateral, and two oblique views when imaging the elbow.

As with the shoulder, the pediatric patient has ossification centers in the elbow joint that appear and fuse at different ages. It is important to know the sequence of the appearance as well as fusion of these ossification centers in order to identify normal from abnormal findings. The order of appearance can be easily remembered with the mnemonic CRITOE, which represents **C**apitellum, **R**adius, **I**nternal or medial epicondyle, **T**rochlea, **O**lecranon, and **E**xternal or lateral epicondyle **(Figure 7.17)**. The ages that these ossification centers appear are highly variable and differ between individuals; however, a general guide or rule of thumb is to remember the following:

C = 1 year
R = 3 years
I = 5 years
T = 7 years
O = 9 years
E = 11 years

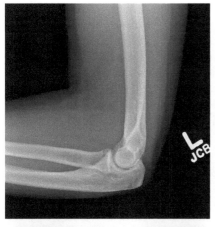
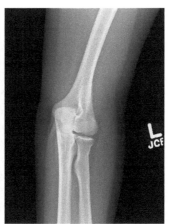
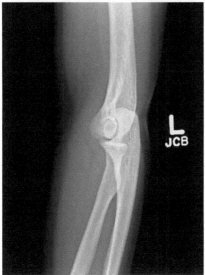

FIGURE 7.16 Three views of a normal elbow study.
Source: Courtesy of Dr. David Begleiter.

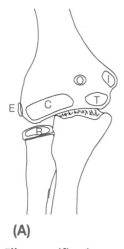
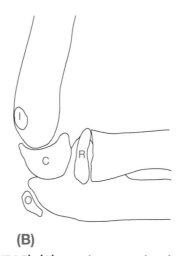

(A)   (B)

FIGURE 7.17 Elbow ossification centers (CRITOE): (A) anterior–posterior view equivalent;
(B) lateral view equivalent.
Source: Drawings by Theresa M. Campo.

Evaluating alignment in the pediatric patient is also important because of the epiphyseal growth plates. The radiocapitellar line is a line drawn through the long axis of the radius that should always point toward the center of the capitellum regardless of the position of the patient since the radius articulates with the capitellum (Figure 7.18). When a dislocation occurs of the radius, the line will not pass through the center of the capitellum. An anterior humeral line is a line that can be drawn on a lateral view along the anterior surface of the humerus and should pass through the middle third of the capitellum (Figure 7.18). With a supracondylar fracture, the anterior humeral line will pass through the anterior third of the capitellum or directly in front of the capitellum due to posterior bending of the distal humeral fragment.

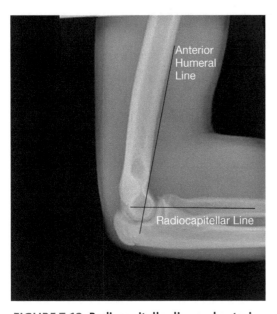

FIGURE 7.18 Radiocapitellar line and anterior humeral line and fracture. Note the anterior humeral line along the anterior aspect of the humerus through the capitellum and the radiocapitellar line traversing the capitellum and intersecting the proximal radius.
Source: Courtesy of Dr. David Begleiter; diagramming by Theresa M. Campo.

Fractures to the distal humerus can involve either the medial condyle or lateral condyle and can be very severe. Fracture of either one or both epicondyles can lead to long-term complications and disability of elbow movement. Fractures can occur anywhere within or above the condyles. Vascular and nerve injuries can occur with significantly displaced condylar fractures due to the brachial artery and median nerve, both lying anteriorly. Supracondylar fractures occurring in children are most commonly caused by a fall on outstretched hand (FOOSH) injury. Table 7.3 provides a description of various condylar fractures.

TABLE 7.3 TYPES OF CONDYLAR FRACTURES

ARTICULAR LOCATION	CONDYLE	FRACTURE LOCATION
Extra-articular	Epicondylar	Medial or lateral epicondyle
	Supracondylar	Above the epicondyle
Intra-articular	Transcondylar	Medial or lateral condyle fracture with fracture plane within the capsule
	Bicondylar	Fracture line splits the medial and lateral epicondyle

Radial head fractures most commonly occur from a FOOSH injury in adults. Occult fractures of the radial head may only be identified by visualization of fat pads. It can be normal to see a very small anterior fat pad located anterior to the coracoid. However, when the anterior fat pad is pushed outward and resembles the sail of a sailboat (known as a sail sign) and/or a posterior fat pad is easily visible, it is due to an effusion caused by leakage of blood from the bone and marrow into the joint. If these occur, an occult fracture must be considered and ruled out with further imaging (Figure 7.19).

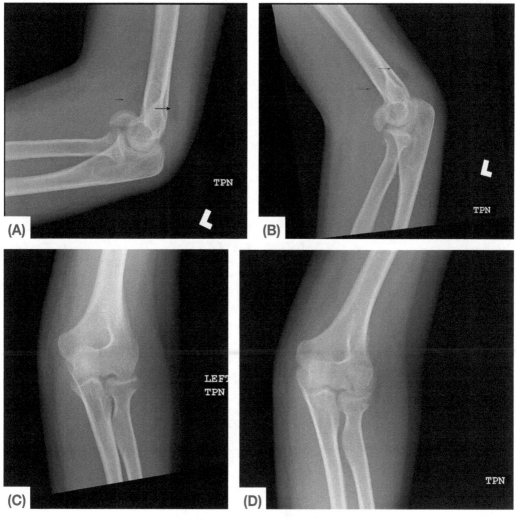

FIGURE 7.19 (A–D) Condylar fracture of the
humerus with an anterior sail sign and posterior fat pad.
Source: Courtesy of Dr. Douglas W. Parrillo; diagramming by Theresa M. Campo.

RADIUS AND ULNA

A distal radial fracture may occur solely or may be associated with dislocation of the distal radioulnar joint. This is commonly known as an Essex–Lopresti fracture (Figure 7.20). If the proximal third of the ulna is fractured with an associated dislocation of the radial head, this is known as a Monteggia fracture (Figure 7.21). The radius and ulna may be fractured anywhere along the shaft of one or both of these bones. Injury may result from either a direct blow to the posterior ulna or a fall with forceful pronation of the forearm. Radial head displacement into the antecubital fossa, elbow pain, and tenderness may be seen on clinical evaluation.

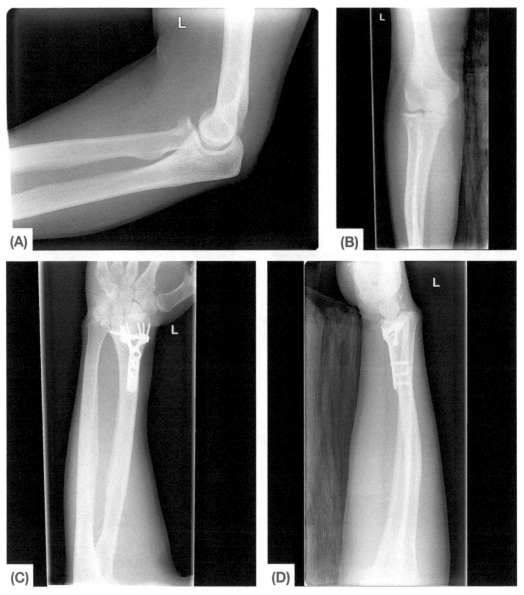

FIGURE 7.20 (A–D) Essex–Lopresti fracture.
Source: Courtesy of Dr. Henry Knipe Radiopaedia.org.

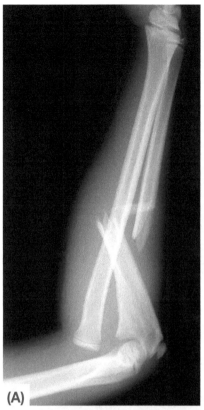

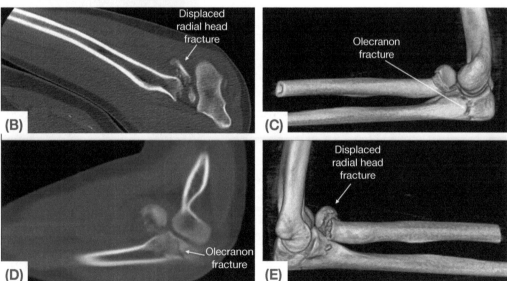

**FIGURE 7.21 (A) Monteggia fracture on radiograph;
(B–E) Monteggia fracture on CT scan with 3D reconstruction.**

Source: (A) Reprinted with permission from Medscape Drugs & Diseases (http://emedicine.medscape.com), 2016.
Available at http://emedicine.medscape.com/article/1231438-overview; (B-E) With permission from Beutel, B. G.,
Klifto, C. S., & Chu, A. (2014). Percutaneous reduction and flexible intramedullary nailing for Monteggia fracture in a
skeletally mature patient. *International Journal of Surgery Case Reports, 5*(12), 1261–1264. https://doi.org/10.1016
/j.ijscr.2014.11.057

A Galeazzi fracture occurs when the proximal radius is fractured and associated with either subluxation or dislocation of the distal ulna (**Figure 7.22**). Barton's fracture occurs when there is displacement of the articular lip of the distal radius that may be associated with a carpal subluxation. A chauffeur's fracture—named during the era of crank automobiles, also known as a Hutchinson fracture—occurs when there is an intra-articular fracture of the radial styloid (**Figure 7.23**). A Colles fracture is when the fracture fragment of the distal radius is dorsally displaced with volar apex angulation (**Figure 7.24**). This fracture most often occurs from a FOOSH injury in elderly females. Approximately 50% of Colles fractures occur with an associated ulnar styloid fracture. When there is a distal radial fracture with volar displacement, it is known as a Smith fracture.

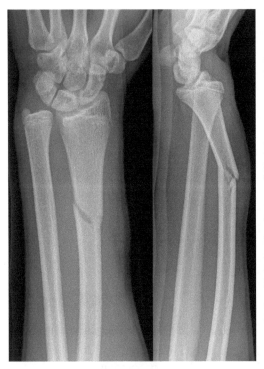

FIGURE 7.22 Galeazzi fracture.
Source: Courtesy of Hellerhoff/Wikipedia Commons.

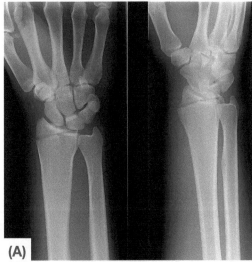

(A)

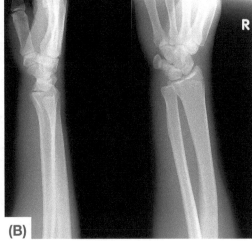

(B)

FIGURE 7.23 (A,B) Chauffeur's fracture.
Source: Copyright 2016 Dr. Alexandra Stanislavsky.
Image courtesy of Dr. Alexandra Stanislavsky and
Radiopaedia.org. Used under license.

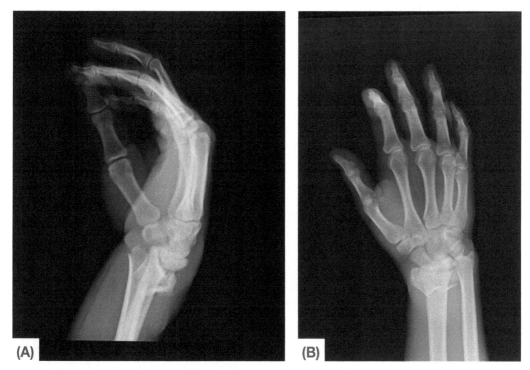

(A) **(B)**

FIGURE 7.24 (A,B) Colles fracture.
Source: Courtesy of Dr. Douglas W. Parrillo.

Long-bone fractures in children that do not penetrate or break through the bony cortex are referred to as greenstick fractures. There are three types of greenstick fractures: transverse fractures occurring only halfway through the bone; torus or buckle fractures where the cortex of the bone buckles and becomes overlapping; and bowing-bent bone when there is no identifiable bony cortex disruption but bowing of the bone is visualized (Figure 7.25).

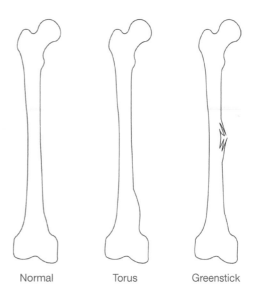

Normal   Torus   Greenstick

FIGURE 7.25 Types of greenstick fractures.
Source: Drawing by Ocean City High School student.

CARPALS

Fractures may occur to any of the carpal bones; however, they are less frequently seen in comparison with metacarpal fractures and distal radius and ulna fractures. Carpal injuries are more commonly associated with separation and dislocation; in addition, fractures to the metacarpals and phalanges occur more frequently than fractures and dislocations of the carpal bones.

A triquetral fracture is the second most common carpal fracture, with scaphoid fracture being the most common. In this type of fracture, there is bone avulsion from the dorsal surface that is best viewed in the lateral view of the hand. Noting any soft tissue abnormalities of the dorsal wrist can also aid in identification of this fracture (Figure 7.26).

Scaphoid fractures, the most common carpal fractures, can be difficult to identify on radiographs (Figure 7.27). Obtaining a scaphoid view of the wrist may aid in identification along with assessing for tenderness in the anatomical snuff box region of the hand. This injury occurs with extreme dorsiflexion of the wrist and ulnar deviation. This type of fracture rarely occurs in children.

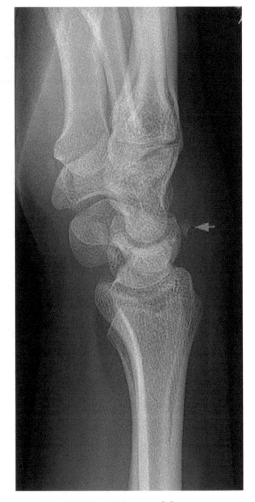

FIGURE 7.26 Triquetral fracture.
Source: **Courtesy of Hellerhoff/Wikipedia Commons.**

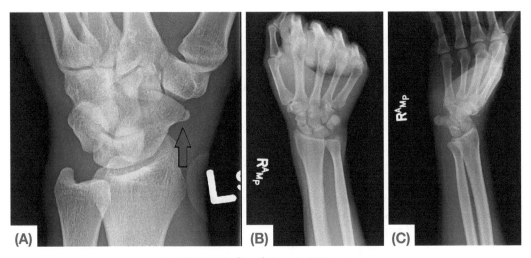

(A)   (B)   (C)

FIGURE 7.27 (A–C) Scaphoid fracture.
Source: **Courtesy of Dr. Douglas W. Parrillo.**

METACARPALS

One of the more common fractures of the hand is a boxer's fracture. This occurs during a punch-type injury or close-fisted impact, causing a fracture to the fifth metacarpal neck with volar displacement of the head of the metacarpal. Boxer's fractures may also involve the fourth metacarpal (Figure 7.28). These can become problematic injuries if

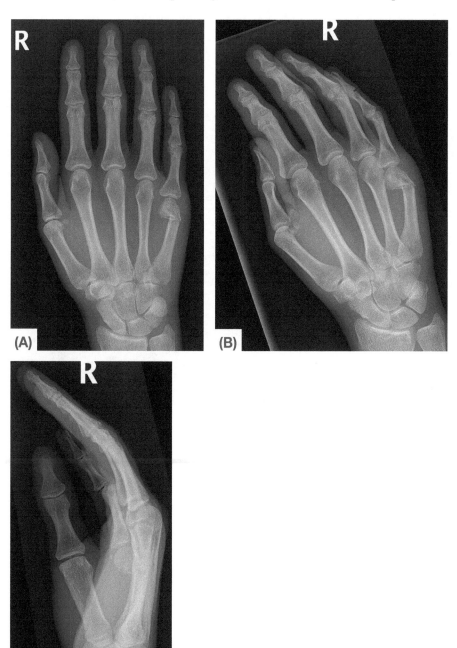

FIGURE 7.28 (A–C) Boxer's fracture.
Source: Copyright 2016 Dr Henry Knipe. Image courtesy of Dr. Henry Knipe and Radiopaedia.org. Used under license.

there is open skin caused by a punch to another person's mouth with bacterial contamination from saliva. It is imperative that any punch injury with a bite and contamination from saliva or mucus be treated as an open fracture with antibiotic prophylaxis combined with close monitoring and orthopedic follow-up.

A Bennett's fracture is an intra-articular fracture—dislocation of the base of the first metacarpal. The separating triangular fragment most commonly dislocates dorsally **(Figure 7.29)**. This type of fracture occurs from axial loading and most commonly occurs from a fight injury. Transverse or oblique are other common metacarpal fractures that may involve one or multiple metacarpals.

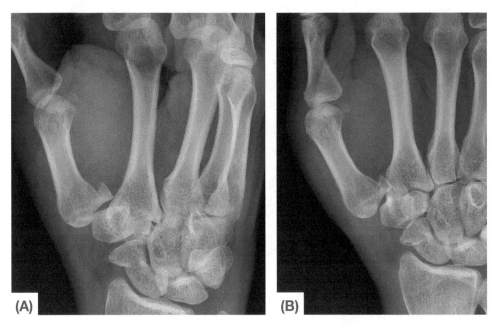

FIGURE 7.29 (A,B) Bennett's fracture.
Source: Copyright 2016 Dr. Maulik S. Patel. Image courtesy of Dr. Maulik S. Patel and Radiopaedia.org.
Used under license.

PHALANGES

Fractures to the phalanges can be caused by crush injuries, jamming of the finger or fingers, or from direct trauma. Fractures to the distal phalanx need to be evaluated for possible nail plate and/or nail bed injury. Comminuted fractures of the tuft of the distal phalanx from a crushing injury may result in partial or full amputation of the distal finger **(Figure 7.30)**.

Dislocations/Subluxations/Separations

Articular surfaces of bones within joints are kept in place by ligaments and cartilage. When the alignment of the adjacent bones is not maintained or they have lost complete contact with each other, then subluxation or dislocation occurs. With subluxation, the articular surface of one bone maintains contact with the articular surface of the adjacent bone. Although the bones are not in complete alignment, they have not lost contact with each other. When a dislocation occurs, the articular surface of one bone loses complete contact with the other, causing a complete disarticulation.

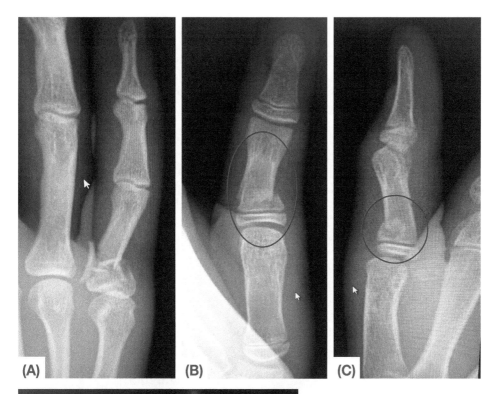

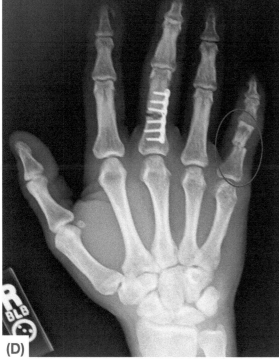

FIGURE 7.30 Phalange fracture: (A) Fracture at the base of the fifth proximal phalanx; (B,C) fracture to the middle phalanx; (D) midshaft fracture of fifth proximal phalanx. Note the appliance to the third proximal phalanx.
Source: Courtesy of Kyle Deuter.

SHOULDER

Dislocations occurring in the shoulder are most commonly anterior, posterior, or inferior. For the purposes of this book, we will only discuss anterior and posterior dislocations, as inferior dislocations are less common. Anterior dislocations are most common, with posterior dislocation occurring in approximately 3% of all cases. Shoulder dislocations are the most commonly occurring due to the incredible range of motion and the anatomical structures that allow for such motion.

When evaluating any film, it is important to have an image in your mind of the normal anatomy. This is helpful when identifying dislocations of the shoulder. Visualize that the humeral head is sitting adjacent to the glenoid if the humeral head is shifted forward or anteriorly; it changes the appearance of the humeral head and proximal end of the humerus on radiograph. In the AP view, the head of the humerus will be under the coracoid and displaced toward the coracoid on the "Y" view. More than 95% of shoulder dislocation occurs anteriorly, with the displacement of the humeral head anterior to the glenoid cavity.

There are four types of anterior dislocations: subcoracoid, subglenoid, subclavicular, and intrathoracic, with the first two being the most commonly occurring. Anterior dislocations occur when indirect force to the arm is combined with abduction, extension, and external rotation of the arm. They may be accompanied by an impaction fracture of the anterior lip of the humeral head known as a Bankart fracture. Another commonly seen fracture associated with anterior dislocation is the Hill–Sachs defect, which is a fracture to the posterior–lateral aspect of the humeral head. This occurs when the humeral head is struck against the glenoid (Figure 7.31).

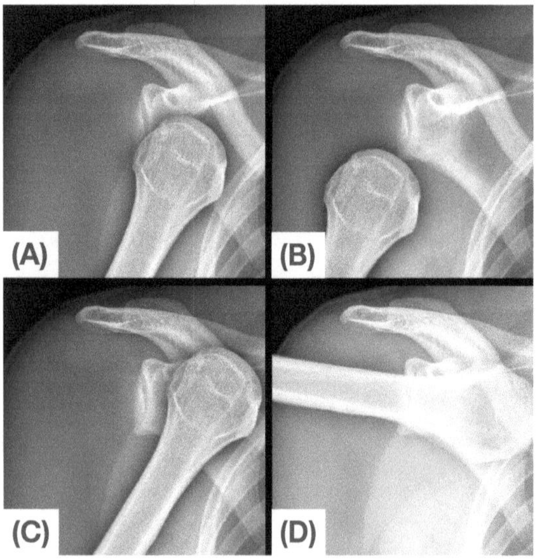

FIGURE 7.31 Four types of anterior dislocation: (A) Subcoracoid; (B) subglenoiod; (C) subclavicular; (D) intrathoracic.
Source: Campo, T. M., & Lafferty, K. A. (Eds.). (2016). *Essential procedures for emergency, urgent, and primary care settings: A companion* (2nd ed.). Springer Publishing.

If the humeral head is shifted backward and is facing posteriorly, again it changes the appearance of the humerus on a radiograph. With a posterior dislocation, the humeral head and proximal end of the humerus will have the appearance of a light bulb, especially in the AP view, and will be outside of the Y of the scapula on the "Y" view. There may be widening of the joint, usually greater than 6 mm, due to the lateral displacement of the humeral head. With approximately 3% of dislocations occurring posteriorly, they are very uncommon. It is caused by internal rotation and adduction from an indirect force. It may occur during a seizure, fall, or electrical/lightning shock. This type of dislocation may be difficult to identify on plain radiographs. Obtaining an axillary view is most beneficial (Figure 7.32).

Injury to the acromioclavicular ligament can cause a separation between the acromium and the clavicle. There are three grades of separation:

Grade I—Minimal displacement of the joint may be visualized on radiograph. There is stretching and possibly partial tearing of the acromioclavicular ligament. This is the most common type of injury to this joint.

Grade II—The acromioclavicular ligament is completely torn but the coracoclavicular ligaments remain intact. This may be apparent on the radiographs as a widening of the acromioclavicular space. However, it may not be obvious during a physical exam.

Grade III—Complete separation of the joint occurs when the acromioclavicular and coracoclavicular ligaments are torn and there is damage to the surrounding capsule. This will be an obvious finding on the radiograph with widening of the acromioclavicular space. Clinically, a bump on the shoulder may be palpated due to the clavicle being pushed upward while the weight of the arm causes the shoulder to fall (Figure 7.33).

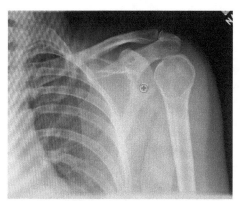
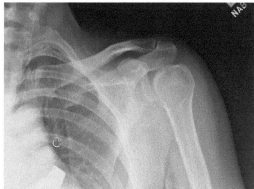
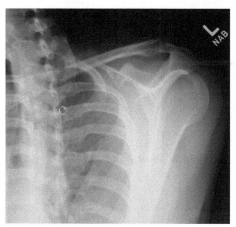

FIGURE 7.32 **Three views demonstrating a posterior dislocation.**
Source: Theresa M. Campo.

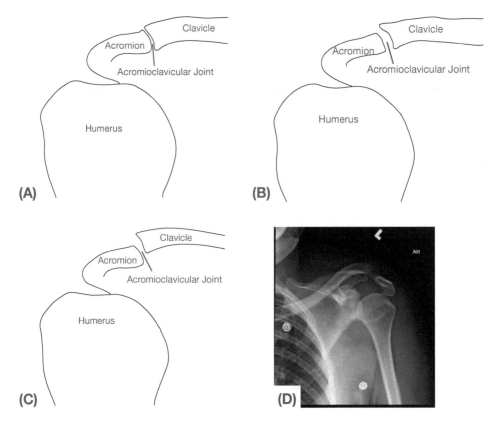

FIGURE 7.33 **Three grades of acromioclavicular (AC) separation: (A) Grade I; (B) grade II; (C) grade III; (D) grade III AC separation on radiograph.**
Source: Drawings courtesy of Theresa M. Campo. Image courtesy of Dr. Douglas W. Parrillo.

ELBOW

The elbow is a large hinge joint that has two articulations. The first articulation is formed between the humerus and the ulna, which allows for flexion and extension. The second articulation is between the radius and humerus, which allows for supination and pronation. The elbow is stabilized by distinctive bony structures and ligaments that protect the joint from varying degrees of force. It takes a great deal of force to cause a dislocation. For this reason, there are usually accompanying fractures of the radial head and coranoid process.

Approximately 90% of elbow dislocations occur posteriorly from a FOOSH-type injury. The other 10% of elbow dislocations may be anterior, divergent, medial, or lateral. Anterior dislocations usually occur from a direct blow to the posterior aspect of a flexed elbow and are commonly associated with brachial artery and median nerve injury. Divergent dislocations are extremely rare and caused by high-energy trauma to the elbow. Medial and lateral dislocations occur when the humerus is displaced either medially or laterally. See Figure 7.34 for an example of an elbow dislocation.

Nurse maid's elbow is not a dislocation but a radial head subluxation. Nurse maid's elbow can occur between the ages of 1 to 5 years of age but most commonly occurs between 2 and 3 years of age. The annular ligament becomes torn from the radial head during a sudden pull on the forearm with the arm extended and minimally pronated. The torn annular ligament then slips between the radial head and the capetellum. This injury does not require medical imaging with a plain radiograph unless the mechanism is of a direct blow or other traumatic event. Ultrasound is being used to identify nurse maid's elbow and

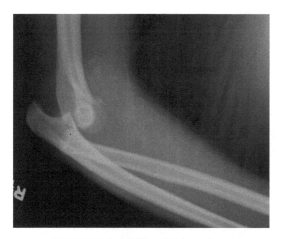

FIGURE 7.34 Elbow dislocation.
Source: Courtesy of Theresa M. Campo.

to confirm reduction of the annular ligament. However, clinical correlation with use of the arm again, following closed reduction, is typically confirmatory.

WRIST

Lunate and perilunate dislocations occur most frequently from a FOOSH but may also occur from a direct blow to the palm of the hand, causing dorsiflexion and ulnar deviation. Perilunate dislocations occur two to three times more frequently than lunate dislocations. Lunate dislocations occur when the lunate displaces volarly and rotates up to 90° from both the capitate and radius. Lunate dislocations are best seen in the lateral view with typical radius—lunate—capitate lines of the bones rotating medially and distally (Figure 7.35). Perilunate dislocations occur when the capitate is displaced from the lunate, most commonly toward the dorsal surface. Perilunate dislocations are also best visualized on the lateral view with the lunate in proper alignment with the radius with accompanying capitate dislocation. The AP view shows crowding of the carpals with overlapping of the proximal and distal rows. Approximately 75% of perilunate dislocations have an associated scaphoid fracture (Figure 7.36).

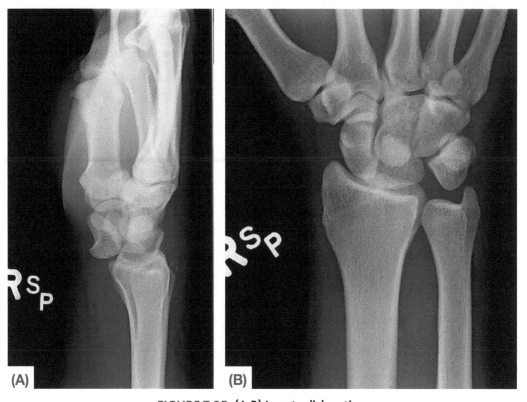

(A)   (B)

FIGURE 7.35 (A,B) Lunate dislocation.
Source: Reprinted by permission of James Heilman, MD, Wikipedian, ER Department Head, East Kootenay Regional Hospital, Clinical Assistant Professor, Department of Emergency Medicine, University of British Columbia.

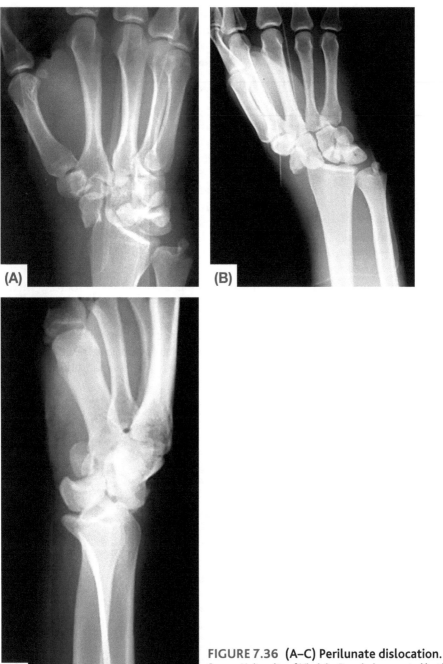

FIGURE 7.36 (A–C) Perilunate dislocation.
Source: University of Virginia. Permission granted by the University of Virginia Department of Radiology and Medical Imaging.

Scapholunate dissociation also occurs with FOOSH injuries. The force of the impact causes rotary subluxation of the scaphoid and results in a gap between the scaphoid and lunate on the AP view. This is known as the Terry Thomas sign.

PHALANGES

Dislocations can occur at any of the phalangeal joints and are considered either simple or complex. In simple dislocations, there is no soft tissue entrapment within the joint. When soft tissue becomes entrapped in the joint, the dislocation is considered to be complex and reduction may be quite difficult. Dislocation of metacarpal phalangeal/interpharlangeal (MCP/IP) joints is described by the specific affected joint and the direction of the distal phalanx.

It is important to note that any fracture or dislocation that is reduced should have a post-reduction radiograph to confirm realignment and reduction. Post-reduction images can also rule in or out an accompanying fracture that was not visible due to the dislocation. Depending on the extent and stability of the fracture and/or dislocation, the post-reduction film may need to occur either before or after a splint or cast has been applied.

BONE LESIONS

When evaluating the bone structures, growths of a benign or malignant etiology may be identified. When evaluating a bony lesion on radiograph, one should consider if the margins are ill-defined, well-defined, or sclerotic. Next, consider the patient's age and, finally, where the lesion is located. Well-defined and sclerotic lesions in individuals younger than 40 years of age are usually benign with the exception of a well-defined chondrosarcoma, which occurs most often between the ages of 20 and 40 years. Ill-defined lytic lesions or any new bony lesions after the age of 40 years are highly suspicious for malignancy or metastasis and should have further evaluation (Figure 7.37).

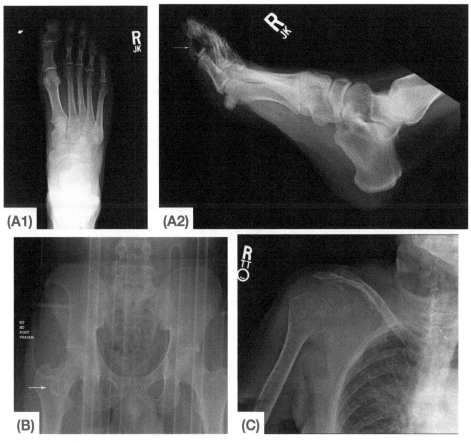

FIGURE 7.37 (A1) Ill-defined and (A2) well-defined lytic lesion great toe;
(B) rim sclerotic lesion enchondroma right femur; (C) sclerotic lesions.
Source: Courtesy of Dr. Douglas W. Parrillo; diagramming by Theresa M. Campo.

CONCLUSION

Falls and direct trauma are the most common causes of injury to the upper extremities. There are many terms used to identify types of fractures and dislocations. The important thing to remember is to clearly describe, using correct anatomical terminology, what is visualized on an image and not become overly concerned about the "proper name" of a fracture or dislocation. Proper identification of the bone, area of the bone, and type of fracture is all that is needed to discuss your findings with colleagues and radiologists. The ability to properly identify normal anatomical structures is paramount to understanding what you are visualizing on a radiograph and why. Always match the mechanism of injury with the findings themselves. If a mechanism does not match the findings, then suspicion for abuse is necessary and warranted. Keep looking at upper extremity films to improve your interpretation proficiency and confidence. Have fun!

RESOURCES

Au-Yong, I., Au-Yong, A., & Broderick, N. (2010). *On-call x-rays made easy*. Churchill Livingstone, Elsevier.

Beutel, B. G., Klifto, S., & Chu, A. (2014). Percutaneous reduction and flexible intramedullary nailing for monteggia fracture in a skeletally mature patient. *International Journal of Surgery Case Reports, 5*(12), 1261–1264. https://doi.org/10.1016/j.ijscr.2014.11.057

Campo, T., & Lafferty, K. A. (2021). *Essential procedures for emergency, urgent, and primary care settings* (3rd ed.). Springer Publishing Company.

Daffner, R. H. (2014). Musculoskeletal imaging. In R. H. Daffner & M. S. Hartman (Eds.), *Clinical radiology: The essentials* (4th ed., pp. 353–429). Wolters Kluwer/Lippincott Williams & Wilkins.

Hahn, B. (2022). *Imaging of clavicular fractures and dislocations*. Medscape. retrieved from https://emedicine.medscape.com/article/398799-overview

Helms, C. A., & Vinson, E. N. (2018). Skeletal trauma. In W. E. Brant & C. A. Helms (Eds.), *Fundamentals of diagnostic radiology* (5th ed., pp. 1015–1042). Wolters Kluwer/Lippincott Williams & Wilkins.

Herring, W. (2016). *Learning radiology: Recognizing the basics* (3rd ed., pp. 240–253). Elsevier.

Kuntz, A. F., Lai, W. S., Norton, P. T., Yao, L. L., & Gay, S. B. *Skeletal trauma*. https://introductiontoradiology.net/courses/rad/ext/

McKinnis, L. N. (2020). *Fundamentals of musculoskeletal imaging* (5th ed.). F. A. Davis.

Nunn, H., & Nunn, D. (n.d.). *Norwich image interpretation course*. http://www.imageinterpretation.co.uk

Schmidt, J. C. (2020). *Scapula (shoulder blade) fracture management in the emergency department*. Medscape. https://emedicine.medscape.com/article/826084-overview

CHAPTER 8

Basic Interpretation of Long Bone—Lower Extremity Radiographs

Radiographs of long bones, whether of the upper extremity or the lower extremity, are usually performed as a result of a traumatic injury. However, pain, swelling, and/or redness may also be indications for obtaining radiographs to rule out abnormal growth, infection, bursitis, or foreign body. Plain radiographs of long bones are beneficial in identifying fractures, subluxation, dislocation, and soft tissue swelling in traumatic injuries, but are also beneficial in identifying abnormal bone growths for nontraumatic signs and symptoms.

In this chapter, normal findings on plain radiographs are discussed, as well as common findings in adults and children. When interpreting long-bone radiographs, the knowledge of normal anatomical structures is imperative. We discuss not only the anatomical structures on the radiographs but also normal alignment of joint structures and normal variants that may be seen.

NORMAL

Before ordering any plain radiographs of long bones or joints, it is important to review some of the rules discussed in earlier chapters. When evaluating the lower extremity, it is important to not only assess the area of complaint but also to examine the joint above and below the affected area. For instance, if the patient complains of an injury to the shin, the radiological study should include the knee as well as the ankle. Routine studies should include a minimum of two views, with most studies having three views or more depending on the area in question.

Plain radiographs are excellent in identifying bony abnormalities such as fractures. Even though radiographs are not the best modality for evaluating soft tissue structures, such as cartilage, muscle, tendons, and ligaments that make up a particular joint, plain films can identify changes within the alignment of the bones making up the joint and show edema that is inflammatory in nature, resulting from an occult bone fracture or from other causes of traumatic injury.

Lower extremity radiographs include the pelvis, hip, knee, ankle, metatarsal, and phalangeal joints, as well as the bones that make up these joints; that is, the pelvic bones, femur, tibia, fibula, patella, tarsals, metatarsals, and phalanges. Each joint in each bone has a different appearance as well as function. Any abnormalities can cause a loss of normal function and use of the lower extremity. As discussed in the previous chapter, there are five types of bones in the body; these can be seen in Table 7.1 of Chapter 7. When evaluating bone images, it is important to visualize the cortical margins in order to identify any abnormalities.

The *ABCs* of interpretation can be utilized for systematic assessment of the lower extremity. *A* is for *adequacy* and *alignment*. As stated in previous chapters, *A*dequacy of the film is of the utmost importance when evaluating any radiographs. Knowledge of proper *A*lignment, which refers to the bone itself and its orientation within the joint, allows the viewer to identify subtle abnormalities. *B* is for *bones* and refers to the evaluation of all components of the bone in the respective study. Cortical margins and borders should be evaluated for any disruption or lack of continuity indicative of a fracture. Scan for any abnormal growths or lesions, which may appear as densities or opacities on the radiograph image. *C* stands for *cartilage* and joints, which can be evaluated for abnormalities by visualizing the joint space. Loss of the normal joint space or asymmetry may be indicative of a crush injury or a sign of degenerative joint disease. Bulging or displacement of normal structures in the lower extremity may be indicative of a fracture or a joint effusion. In the mnemonic, *s* is for *soft* tissues, which can show signs of trauma through abnormal joint effusion or edema. Scan for radiopaque foreign bodies within the bone and soft tissues.

DESCRIBING FRACTURES

Bone fractures can result from injury or pathology. Describe fractures using correct anatomical terminology when interpreting findings. Remember, fracture lines or patterns may be transverse, oblique, spiral, comminuted, impacted, avulsed, compressed, or depressed **(Figure 8.1)**. Fractures may only involve one side of the bone, both sides, or go completely through the bone itself.

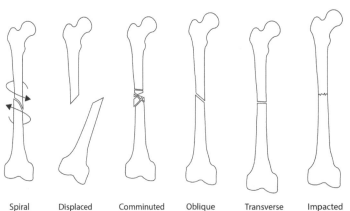

Spiral   Displaced   Comminuted   Oblique   Transverse   Impacted

FIGURE 8.1 Fracture lines or patterns.
Source: Drawing by Ocean City High School student.

Fractures may affect a single bone or be noted in multiple bones; multiple fractures may occur in the same bone but in different areas. Bone fragments are also described as displaced or nondisplaced. When a bone fragment is 100% displaced, there is shortening along with overlapping of the bone fragments, referred to as a bayonet deformity **(Figure 8.2)**. When bone fragments are out of alignment with each other, they are angulated. Angulation is the angle between the longitudinal axis of the main fracture fragment with that of the other fragment. Significant angulation requires reduction and realignment of the bone fragments for proper healing. If a fracture line enters the joint space, it is referred to as an intra-articular fracture **(Figure 8.3)**.

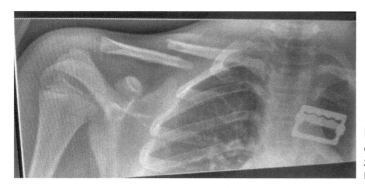

FIGURE 8.2 Bayonet deformity.
Source: Courtesy of Dr. David Begleiter.

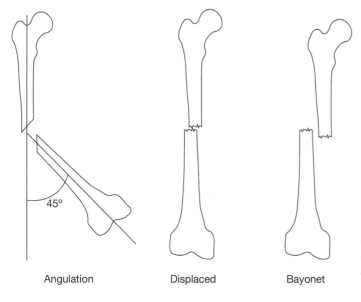

Angulation   Displaced   Bayonet

FIGURE 8.3 Angulation, displacement, and bayonet deformity.
Source: Drawing by Ocean City High School student.

A stress fracture can occur with repetitive loading beyond the bone's tolerance. An avulsion fracture occurs when there is a forcible muscular contraction affecting the tendinous attachment and a piece of bone is pulled off the main structure.

PEDIATRIC CONSIDERATIONS

Consideration needs to be given when interpreting pediatric radiographs. Pediatric bones are more fibrous and less crystalline (calcified) than adult bones. They are enclosed in a sheet of strong fibrous periosteum and have epiphyseal growth plates, which are zones of weakness. Because of these differences, children tend to have incomplete fractures because the bone ends do not separate as they do in adults due to the strong periosteal sleeve in children. The most common types of fractures in the pediatric patient are elastic deformation, bowing deformation, torus or buckle fracture, greenstick fracture, Salter–Harris fracture, stress injury, and avulsion injury (Figure 8.4).

Pediatric bones have epiphyseal growth plates where new osteoclast formation allows the bones to grow. In mature adult bones the epiphyseal growth plates become ossified and new growth no longer occurs. The epiphyseal growth plate is a zone of weakness, which can make fracture, separation, and slipping of the growth plate more common in the pediatric patient.

When a fracture occurs within or around the growth plate, growth disturbances can occur resulting in a loss of function and further growth.

There are five types of growth plate fractures that that make up the Salter–Harris classification system based on abnormalities involving the metaphysis, epiphysis, and/or diaphysis. A Salter I fracture is a separation of the growth plate without involvement of the metaphysis or the epiphysis. A Salter II fracture occurs across the growth plate but with a small fragment of metaphysis remaining attached to the epiphysis. A fracture across the growth plate with extension of the fracture line across the epiphysis is known as a Salter III fracture. When the fracture line traverses the epiphysis and part of the metaphysis, this is known as a Salter IV fracture. Finally, when there is damage to both the epiphysis and the metaphysis from a crush injury, this is known as a Salter V fracture. As you will notice, the

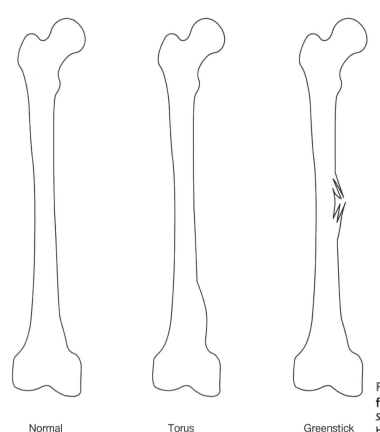

Normal   Torus   Greenstick

FIGURE 8.4 **Pediatric fracture.**
Source: **Drawing by Ocean City High School student.**

severity of the injury increases with the designated number of the Salter–Harris fracture (Figure 8.5). An easy mnemonic to remember the Salter classification is *SALTR*, where *S* refers to a *slip* as in a Salter I, *A* refers to the fracture noted *above* or proximal to the epiphyseal plate, L refers to a fracture *below* or distal to the epiphyseal plate, *T* is a fracture line extending *through* the epiphyseal plate including both the epiphysis and metaphysis, and *R* refers to *crush*.

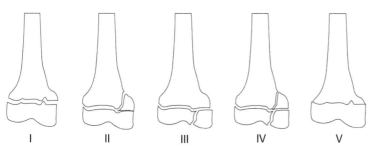

I   II   III   IV   V

FIGURE 8.5 Five types of Salter–Harris fractures.
Source: Drawing by Ocean City High School student.

ABNORMALITIES OF THE LOWER EXTREMITY

Pelvis

The pelvis is composed of eight bones—the ilium (2), ischium (2), pubis (2), the sacrum, and the coccyx—that make up three bony rings. The main ring includes the sacroiliac joints and the symphysis pubis, and the two smaller rings are made up of the pubis and ischial bones (Figure 8.6).

When imaging the pelvis, order an anterior–posterior (AP) view. When obtaining a pelvic image, it is important that the femurs are internally rotated on the AP view for visualization of the femoral neck. However, anterior and posterior oblique views can also be done since a true lateral is of no benefit. Additional views for further evaluation of the pelvis include the frog leg or frog lateral view.

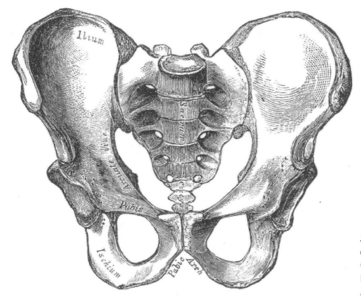

FIGURE 8.6 Pelvic anatomy.
Source: Gray, H. (1918). *Anatomy of the human body.* Henry Vandyke Cater (illustrator). Lea and Febiger Publishers. https://en.wikipedia.org /wiki/Pelvis#/media/File:Gray241.png

Evaluating plain films of the pelvis and hips can be diagnostically challenging. CT scanning may be required if plain films do not show abnormalities yet there is a strong suspicion of an occult or complex fracture, or to determine the degree of displacement and soft tissue injury. Pelvic fractures carry a high risk of mortality due to hemorrhage.

When scanning a pelvic radiograph, check alignment within the joints, symmetry, cortical breaks, and joint spaces (sacroiliac, hip, symphysis pubis). Scan all aspects of the pelvis including the main ring, the two small rings, the two sacroiliac joints, symphysis pubis, sacral foramina, and the acetabular region (Figure 8.7). Ensure that the ilium and ischium are symmetrical and the main ring is circular with smooth borders. Envision the ilium as ears, the main ring a face, and the ischium as a bow tie. In a normal radiograph all the parts are symmetrical and clear (Figure 8.8).

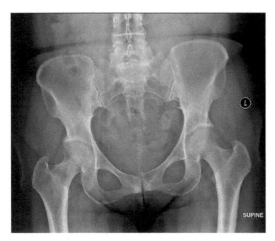

FIGURE 8.7 Normal pelvic radiograph.
Source: Courtesy of Dr. David Begleiter.

When evaluating alignment, note Shenton's line, which is a curved line formed by the top of the obturator foramina in the inner side of the neck of the femur (Figure 8.9). Shenton's line is used to determine the relationship of the head of the femur with the acetabulum. If the line is broken or is disrupted, then a fracture or congenital luxation should be suspected. Scan the bones and joints of the pelvis for normal structure and joint spaces. Evaluate the inner and outer cortices of the main ring as well as the formation of the obturator foramina of the two small rings for disruption of the bony cortex. Scan the alignment of the superior surfaces of the symphysis pubis body. The sacral foramina should

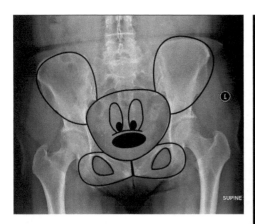

FIGURE 8.8 Envisioning symmetry of the ilium and ischium and smooth borders of the main ring.
Source: Courtesy of Dr. David Begleiter; diagramming by Theresa M. Campo.

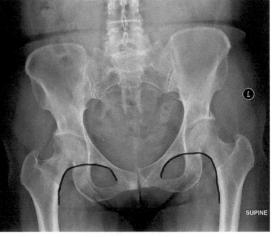

FIGURE 8.9 Shenton's line.
Source: Courtesy of Dr. David Begleiter; diagramming by Theresa M. Campo.

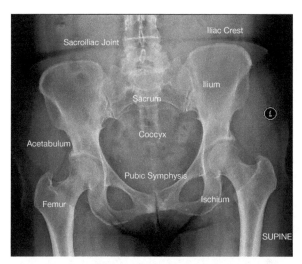

FIGURE 8.10 Pelvic radiograph with marking of structures.
Source: Courtesy of Dr. David Begleiter; diagramming by Theresa M. Campo.

be evaluated for any disruption of the smooth arcuate lines, indicating a fracture, and compare the arcs. The acetabular region should be evaluated for any gross abnormalities; if any are identified, views of the hip should be obtained for further evaluation. See **Figure 8.10** for marked structures.

Assess the symphysis pubis for alignment of the superior surfaces of the pubic bone body. The symphysis pubis width can be up to 10 mm in children but should never be more than 5 mm in adults. The superior cortices of the superior pubic rami should align. The ischial-pubic synchondrosis may present as being irregular and asymmetrical during development until approximately the age of 12 years. The sacroiliac joints may appear normally wide in adolescents, but in adults, they should not be more than 2 to 4 mm in width.

Disruptions in the bone cortex and joint space of the pelvis may not only occur on one side but may also occur in another area due to the nature of the pelvis and its three bone rings. If the main pelvic ring is broken into two areas, then it is considered unstable with the risk of hemorrhage and shock. This injury may also be accompanied by bladder rupture and urethral injury, requiring careful evaluation of the urethra with a retrograde urethrogram prior to any urinary catheterization. Avulsion injuries can be common in the adolescent age group and can be easily missed. Frequent sites for avulsion injuries are the anterior superior iliac spine, anterior inferior iliac spine, and the ischial tuberosity. When there was increased force, complex fractures should be considered, particularly when the sacrum or iliac wing is involved.

Pelvic Fractures

A straddle injury from force against the perineum can result in fracture of the pubic rami bilaterally with the central fragment being displaced superiorly. This may be accompanied by an acetabulum fracture associated with dislocation, which is usually posterior.

Vertical shearing may result in a vertical, unilateral fracture of the pelvic rami with a vertical fracture of the sacral foramina on the same side. This may cause disruption of the sacroiliac joints and possibly fracture to the ilium, paralleling the sacroiliac joint.

A Malgaigne fracture occurs when there is an articular or para-articular fracture of the sacroiliac joint and ipsilateral ischiopubic rami. The clinician will observe shortening of the ipsilateral lower extremity (**Figure 8.11**).

Avulsion fractures can also occur within the pelvis and be easily missed. Common areas of avulsion injury are the inferior and superior anterior iliac spines and the ischial tuberosity. These injuries are usually sport related, caused by the sudden strong contraction of large muscles, and seen in sprinters, gymnasts, cheerleaders, and track and field athletes (sprinters, jumpers, etc.).

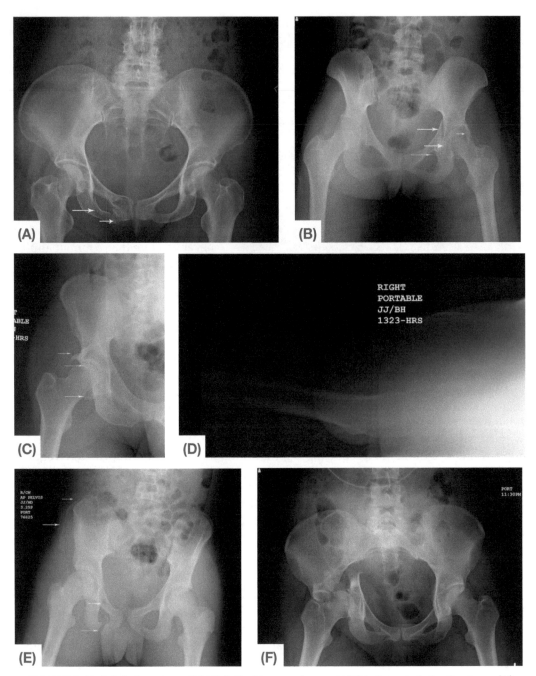

FIGURE 8.11 Pelvic fractures: (A) Right ischium and ramus; (B) left acetabular fracture; (C) comminuted right acetabular fracture; (D) comminuted right acetabular fracture; (E) multiple fractures including alar fracture; and (F) pelvic fracture with displacement.

(continued)

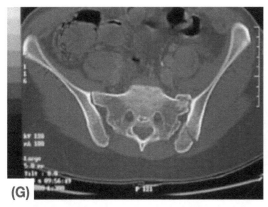

(G)

FIGURE 8.11 *(continued)*
(G) CT scan of a pelvic fracture.
Source: (A–F) Courtesy of Dr. Douglas W. Parrillo;
diagramming by Theresa M. Campo; (G) Reproduced
with permission from Medscape Drugs & Diseases
(https://emedicine.medscape.com/), Unstable Pelvic
Fractures. (2020). https://emedicine.medscape.com
/article/1247426-overview

Sacral Fracture

Sacral fractures are commonly missed in x-ray review and usually occur either vertically or in the transverse plane. Bowel gas may obscure the sacrum, making it difficult to visualize fractures. Sacral fractures may occur on their own or co-occur with pelvic injuries. Examination of the sacrum should begin with the arcuate lines bilaterally to see if they are intact. Disruption of these lines is indicative of a fracture. See **Figure 8.12** regarding the symmetry and asymmetry of arcuate lines.

Anterior force can cause disruption of one or both sacroiliac joints. If there is widening of the symphysis pubis greater than 5 mm with external rotation of the hemi pelvis, this is referred to as the "open book" fracture or injury **(Figure 8.13)**. These injuries are unstable and carry a high risk of hemorrhagic shock. Pelvic dislocation can occur when the sacrum is fractured and there is disruption to both sacroiliac joints with separation of the pubis symphysis. Occult sacral fractures may be present with fracture of the L5 transverse process.

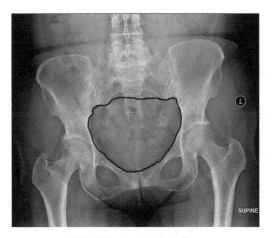

FIGURE 8.12 Arcuate lines.
Source: Courtesy of Dr. David Begleiter; diagramming by
Theresa M. Campo.

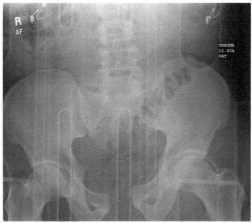

FIGURE 8.13 "Open book" fracture.
Source: Courtesy of Dr. Douglas W. Parrillo.

Hip

The hip is composed of the acetabulum and the femoral head, along with ligaments, the joint capsule, and articular cartilage. When evaluating the hip, AP, lateral, and oblique views are necessary. A one-view pelvis should always be included in the evaluation of the hip **(Figure 8.14)**. The AP view of the hip and pelvis should have the hips internally rotated for full visualization of the femoral neck. Ensure that all views fit the adequacy criteria and

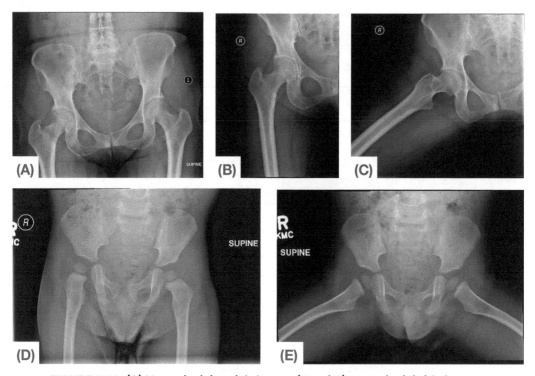

FIGURE 8.14 (A) Normal adult pelvic image; (B and C) normal adult hip images;
and (D and E) normal pediatric hip images.
Source: Courtesy of Dr. David Begleiter.

evaluate the alignment of the bones that make up the hip joint. You will need to evaluate the bone margins for any abnormalities and evaluate the joint itself for signs of effusion or secondary signs of a possible occult fracture. Finally, evaluate the soft tissue for any foreign bodies, gas collection, or other abnormalities (Figure 8.15). If x-rays of the hip and pelvis

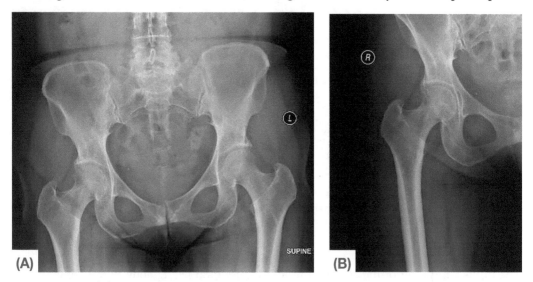

FIGURE 8.15 (A) Evaluation of the pelvis image for symmetry and breaks in the lines of the pelvis; (B) evaluation of the hip image, anterior–posterior view, for alignment of the bony cortex joint space and soft tissue swelling; and

(continued)

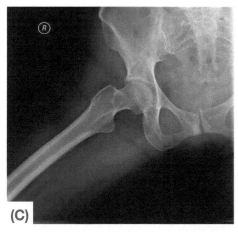

(C)

FIGURE 8.15 (*continued*)
(C) evaluation of the hip image for alignment of the bony cortex, joint space, and soft tissue swelling.
Source: Courtesy of Dr. David Begleiter.

are obtained and show no signs of fracture, it is important to make sure that the patient can ambulate; if not, a CT scan may be necessary to rule out an occult fracture. Fractures of the acetabulum may be difficult to identify but are of utmost importance.

Femur

The proximal femur can be divided into five areas: the femoral head, neck, greater and lesser trochanters, and the proximal femoral shaft **(Figure 8.16)**. Fractures can occur in any of these areas; therefore, it is important to note the location. Subcapital femoral neck fractures occur just below the head of the femur. Transcervical neck fractures occur across the middle of the femoral neck. Intertrochanteric fractures are located at the base of the neck between the greater and lesser trochanters. Fractures can also occur along the greater trochanter, lesser trochanter, or below in the subtrochanteric region **(Figure 8.17)**.

Most commonly, subcapital fractures are impacted or displaced and may be complete or incomplete. They most commonly occur in postmenopausal women from osteroporosis. Avascular necrosis (AVN) of the femoral head results in approximately 20% to 30% of subcapital fractures secondary to the disruption or impingement of the femoral complex arteries. Intertrochanteric femoral fractures generally occur in older adults and are more frequent than subcapital fractures in the aging population.

The femur also has the potential to dislocate either anterior or posterior to the acetabulum. Most dislocations (90%) occur posteriorly from a high-energy force, such as when the knees impact a dashboard during a motor vehicle accident. Assess for a possible posterior rim acetabular fracture, which may accompany a dislocation. The femoral head sits

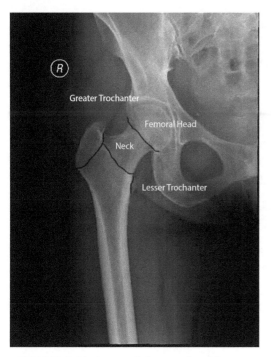

Greater Trochanter

Femoral Head

Neck

Lesser Trochanter

FIGURE 8.16 Areas of the proximal femur.
Source: Courtesy of Dr. David Begleiter; diagramming by Theresa M. Campo.

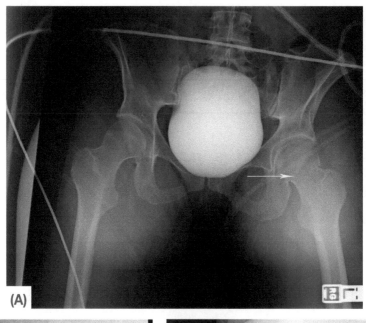

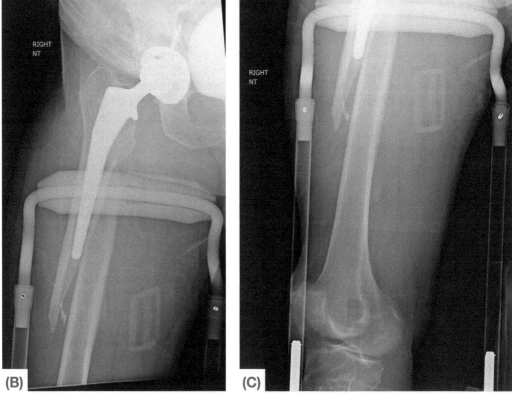

FIGURE 8.17 Different fracture areas of the proximal femur: (A) Subcapital fracture proximal femur; (B and C) proximal femur fracture (note the traction splint).

Source: Courtesy of Dr. Douglas W. Parrillo.

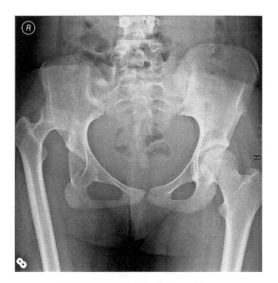

FIGURE 8.18 Hip dislocation.
Source: Reprinted by permission of James Heilman, MD, Wikipedian, ER Department Head, East Kootenay Regional Hospital, Clinical Assistant Professor, Department of Emergency Medicine, University of British Columbia.

lateral and superior to the acetabulum with internal rotation and abduction of the femur, and may appear smaller on the radiographic image secondary to magnification (Figure 8.18).

AVN, also known as osteonecrosis, results from lack of blood supply to the femoral head resulting in bone death (Figure 8.19). AVN is a painful weight-bearing condition that can occur from trauma, prolonged corticosteroid use, alcohol abuse, chemotherapy, sickle-cell disease, or history of a diving and nitrogen toxicity type injury. An MRI may be necessary to visualize the fracture and abnormal bone tissue.

Midshaft femur fractures can occur anywhere along the femoral shaft and may be transverse, oblique, spiral, or comminuted. It takes a great deal of force to cause a fracture in the femur so it is important to ascertain that the mechanism matches the finding on the radiograph. Distal fractures can involve either the medial or lateral condyle of the femur leading up into the shaft (Figure 8.20). These can be complex injuries causing significant soft tissue swelling and the potential for large volume blood loss.

Abnormalities of the hip joint and femur can occur in the pediatric population. A slipped femoral capital epiphysis (SFCE) is a Salter–Harris I fracture and commonly occurs in overweight children and adolescent boys over the 8 years of age. This fracture can occur either

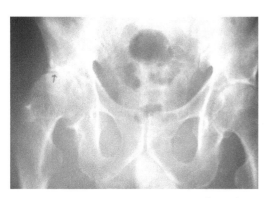

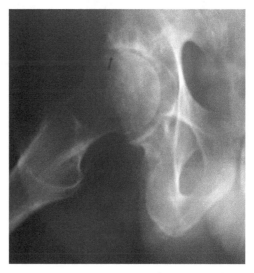

FIGURE 8.19 Avascular necrosis (AVN). Note loss of integrity bony cortex (right image).
Source: Reprinted with permission from Medscape Drugs & Diseases. (2016). http://emedicine.medscape.com. http://emedicine.medscape.com/ article/386808-overview

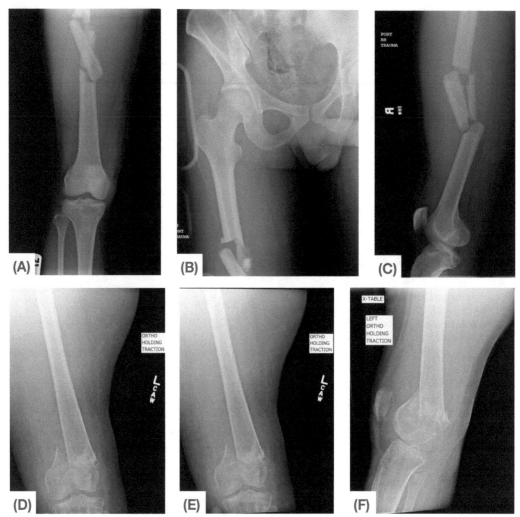

FIGURE 8.20 Medial and lateral condyle fractures. (A–C) Midshaft femur fracture; (D–F) distal femur fracture.
Source: Courtesy of Dr. Douglas W. Parrillo.

unilaterally or bilaterally and may be associated with minor trauma. On a plain film, an SFCE presents as a widening of the epiphyseal plate of the proximal femur. Obtaining a frog leg view may make it easier to identify medial slipping of the epiphyseal plate than on an AP view. To identify this abnormality, draw a line along the lateral femoral neck. If it is not congruent and does not intersect the femoral epiphysis, be suspicious of medial slipping of the epiphyseal plate. See **Figure 8.21** demonstrating an SFCE and the lines demonstrating the abnormality.

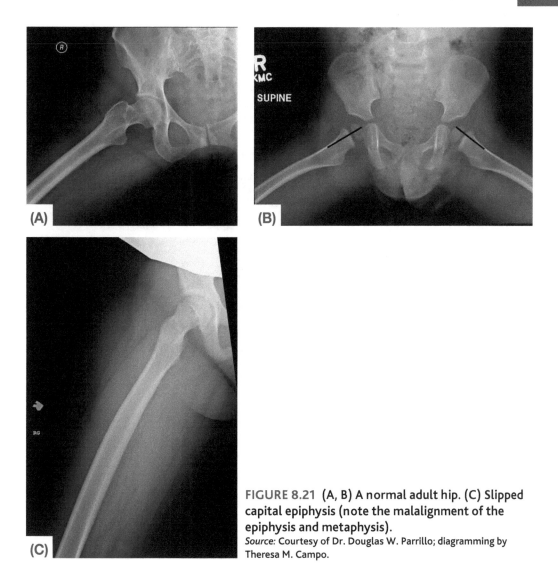

FIGURE 8.21 (A, B) A normal adult hip. (C) Slipped capital epiphysis (note the malalignment of the epiphysis and metaphysis).
Source: Courtesy of Dr. Douglas W. Parrillo; diagramming by Theresa M. Campo.

Osteochondritis dissecans is a condition where bone that lies beneath the cartilage of a joint dies from lack of blood flow. This can occur in numerous places in the body and is labeled based on the area where it is found. Legg–Calve–Perthes disease denotes an osteochondritis occurring at the femoral head. This most commonly occurs in boys younger than the age of 8. On a plain film, the femoral head will appear to have a patchy sclerotic and flattened articular surface resulting from avascular necrosis (Figure 8.22). An MRI may be necessary to visualize this condition.

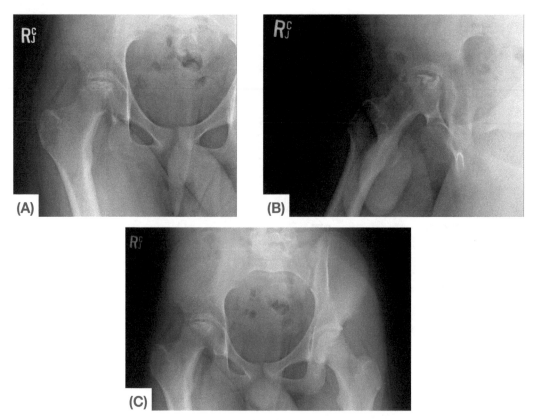

FIGURE 8.22 Legg–Calve–Perthes disease. (A–C) Note the abnormality of the femoral head.
Source: Courtesy of Dr. Douglas W. Parrillo.

Knee

The knee is a large and complex joint with three articulations: medial tibial femoral, lateral tibial femoral, and patellofemoral. Stability of the knee is provided by four ligaments: medial, lateral collateral, anterior, and posterior cruciate ligaments. Evaluation of the knee should include an AP, lateral, and two oblique views (**Figure 8.23**). An additional image, the sunrise or skyline view, may be helpful in evaluating patellar fractures (**Figure 8.24**).

Injuries to the knee are common due to the complexity of the joint, and most commonly involve soft tissue and cartilaginous structures. Radiographs are useful in identifying fractures as well as effusions. However, an MRI is the best modality for evaluating this complex joint.

Knee fractures can result from either a direct blow or from a violent contraction of the quadricep muscle. Obtain a sunrise view if suspicious of an occult and overt fracture of the patella. Patellar fractures may be vertical, horizontal, or comminuted. If a transverse fracture of the patella is suspected or visualized in the AP view, then you should not perform a sunrise view to avoid excessive joint manipulation that can cause displacement. A transverse avulsion patellar fracture can result from violent contraction of the quadricep muscle from sports activities. Transverse avulsion fractures are more common than longitudinal or comminuted patellar fractures. A bipartite patella is a normal variant and can be differentiated from an acute fracture from its rounded margins that don't easily fit together. In contrast, a patellar fracture will look like a piece of a puzzle that fits together visually (**Figure 8.25**).

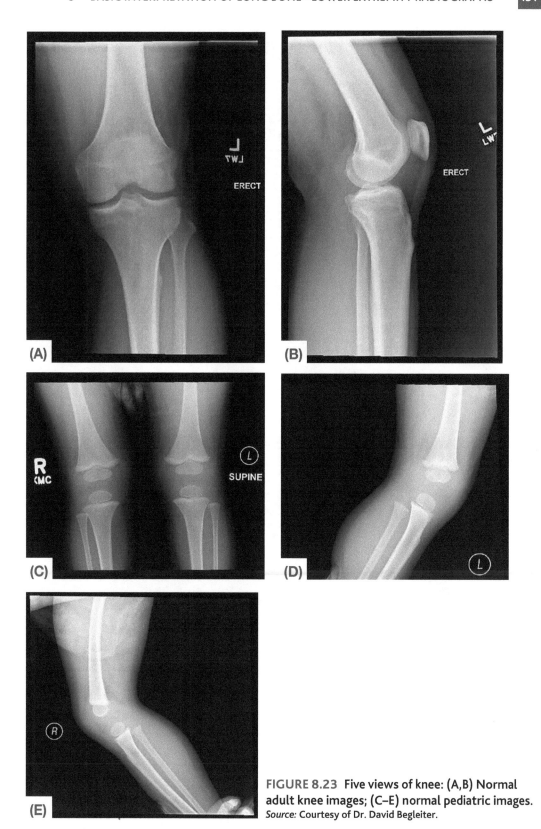

FIGURE 8.23 Five views of knee: (A,B) Normal adult knee images; (C–E) normal pediatric images.
Source: Courtesy of Dr. David Begleiter.

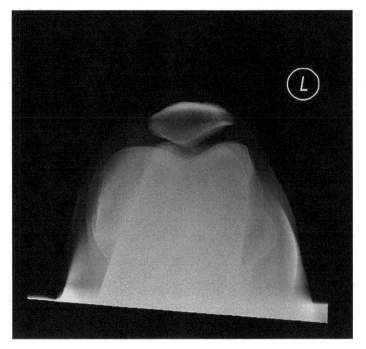

FIGURE 8.24 Sunrise view.
Source: Courtesy of Dr. David Begleiter.

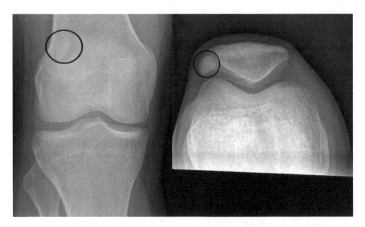

FIGURE 8.25 Bipartite. Note well-corticated area in circles.
Source: Courtesy of Heller Hoff (2016)/Wikipedia Commons; diagramming by Theresa M. Campo.

True dislocations of the knee are rare but usually occur in an anterior translation of the tibia on the femur. Anterior translation is when the tibia displaces anteriorly to the femur. In the case of a true dislocation, consider the possibility of a popliteal artery and/or nerve injury as well as multiple ligamentous tears; these can be diagnosed easily even before a radiograph is obtained **(Figure 8.26)**.

Inflammation of the suprapatellar bursa can cause knee pain and swelling, shifting the position of the anterior and posterior fat pad compartments located posterior to the quadricep tendon in the joint capsule. This corresponding area of the fat pad normally measures less

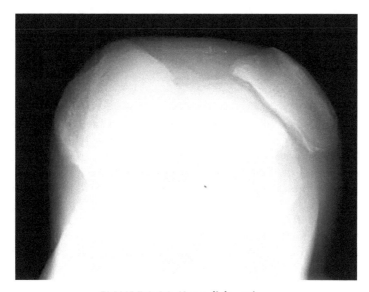

FIGURE 8.26 Knee dislocation.
Source: University of Virginia. Permission granted by the University of Virginia Department of Radiology
and Medical Imaging.

than 5 mm. However, the fat pad can expand and enlarge from a soft tissue injury causing an effusion. Additionally, intraarticular fractures can cause leakage of blood and bone marrow into the joint space, distending the bursa and enlarging the fat pad. Fat lying on top of the fluid is seen radiographically as a fluid–fluid line or density on the lateral view (**Figure 8.27**).

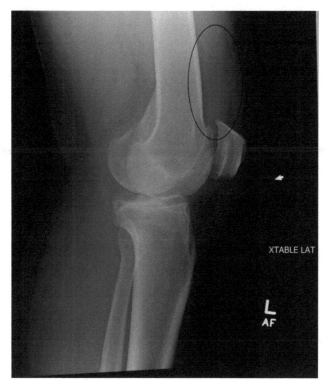

FIGURE 8.27 Knee effusion.
Source: Courtesy of Dr. Douglas W. Parrillo.

Tibia

The tibia plateau is divided into the lateral and medial aspects **(Figure 8.28)**. Fractures of the tibial plateau are commonly labeled as "fender" or "bumper" fractures because they can result from a motor vehicle striking the leg. Tibial plateau fractures commonly occur on the lateral aspect and may be associated with an anterior cruciate ligament (ACL), medial-cruciate ligament (MCL), or medial meniscus injury from valgus stress placed on the knee. Look closely at the tibial plateau because it may be difficult to visualize a fracture if it is not depressed or impacted: a lucent fracture line with increased density may denote impaction or depression. Draw a perpendicular line at the most lateral margin of the femoral condyle and medial cortex of the fibula for alignment. There should not be more than 5 mm of the condyle located laterally **(Figures 8.29** and **8.30)**. If a fracture is not seen, but the suspicion is high for a tibial plateau fracture, obtain a CT scan of the knee.

A Segond fracture is an avulsion of the lateral aspect of the tibial plateau at the attachment of the lateral capsule **(Figure 8.31)**. This injury results from varus stress with internal rotation of the leg, with the knee in a flexed position, that puts excess tension on the lateral capsule and its associated ligaments. This mechanism may also cause an accompanying ACL tear.

Midshaft fractures of the tibia may occur solely or with an accompanying fibula fracture, depending on the mechanism of injury and the force allotted to cause the fracture. Fractures may occur anywhere along the shaft of the tibia and should be matched with the mechanism of injury to rule out abuse as the cause of injury.

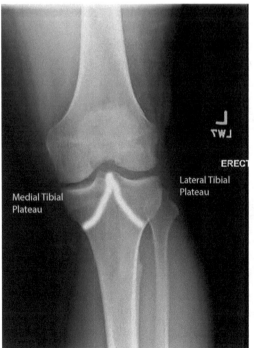

FIGURE 8.28 Medial and lateral aspect tibia plateau.
Source: Courtesy of Dr. David Begleiter; diagramming by Theresa M. Campo.

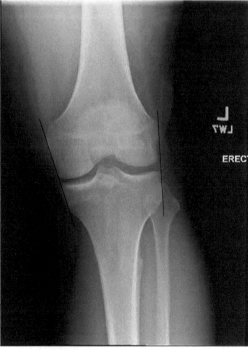

FIGURE 8.29 Medial and lateral lines.
Source: Courtesy of Dr. David Begleiter; diagramming by Theresa M. Campo.

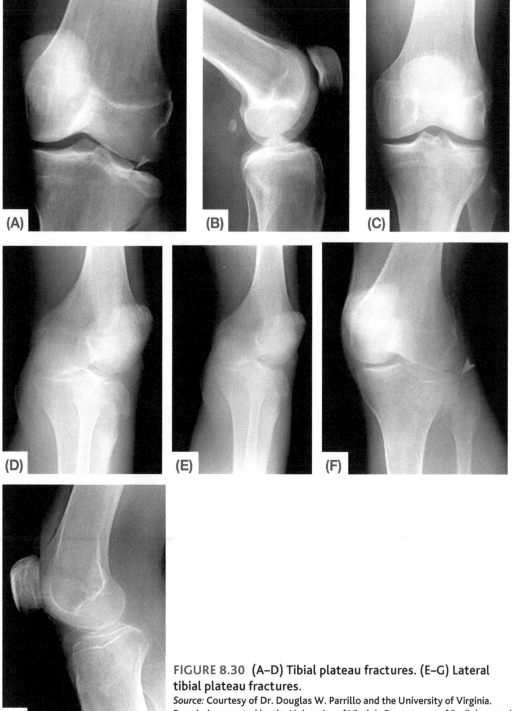

FIGURE 8.30 (A–D) Tibial plateau fractures. (E–G) Lateral tibial plateau fractures.
Source: Courtesy of Dr. Douglas W. Parrillo and the University of Virginia. Permission granted by the University of Virginia Department of Radiology and Medical Imaging.

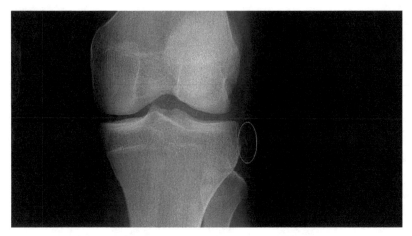

FIGURE 8.31 **Segond fracture.**
Souorce: Courtesy of Ellisbjohns (2009)/Wikipedia Commons.

An avulsion of the lateral margin of the distal tibia is known as a Tillaux fracture (**Figure 8.32**). The mechanism of this injury is abduction and external rotation of the leg. A fracture line vertically extending from the distal articular surface in an upward direction to the lateral cortex of the tibia will be seen on a plain film. Surgery may be required for this injury if there is lateral displacement greater than 2 mm of the fracture fragments distal to the articular surface. Otherwise, if less than 2 mm displacement or no displacement is involved, conservative treatment is usually indicated with closed reduction and immobilization with application of a cast.

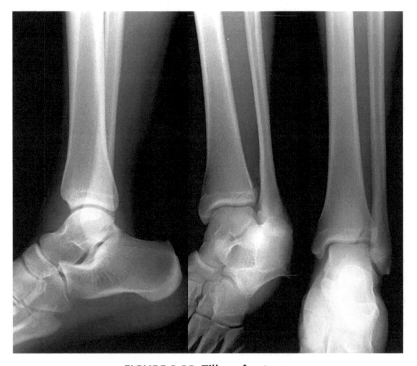

FIGURE 8.32 **Tillaux fracture.**
Source: University of Virginia. Permission granted by the University of Virginia
Department of Radiology and Medical Imaging.

Fibula

Proximal fibula fractures of the head and neck may be associated with tibial plateau fractures or ligamentous injuries to the cruciate or collateral ligaments of the knee. The Maisonneuve fracture occurs when there is strong eversion of the ankle, causing a fracture of the proximal half of the fibula accompanied by fracture of the medial malleolus of the distal tibia and disruption of the tibiofibular syndesmosis; a complete tear may occur (Figure 8.33).

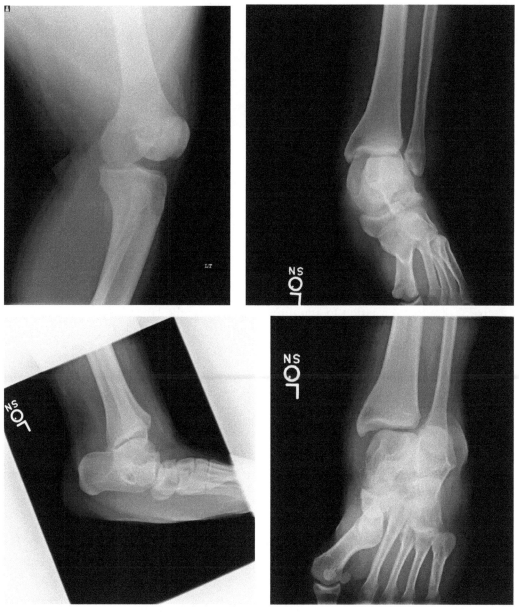

FIGURE 8.33 Maisonneuve fracture.
Source: Courtesy of Dr. Douglas W. Parrillo.

Midshaft fractures of the fibula may occur in conjunction with a midshaft tibia fracture. When examining a plain film of the tibia and fibula, visually trace the margins of both bones in their entirety, looking for any disruptions, lucencies, or densities indicative of multiple fractures.

Osteochondritis of the anterior tibial tuberosity, also known as Osgood Schlatter's disease, occurs in adolescents. This often painful, inflammatory condition usually occurs from repeated trauma to a normal growth zone and ossification center at the tibial tuberosity. This condition can present on a radiographic image with a wide variety of normal variance and may be mistaken for an avulsion fracture (Figure 8.34).

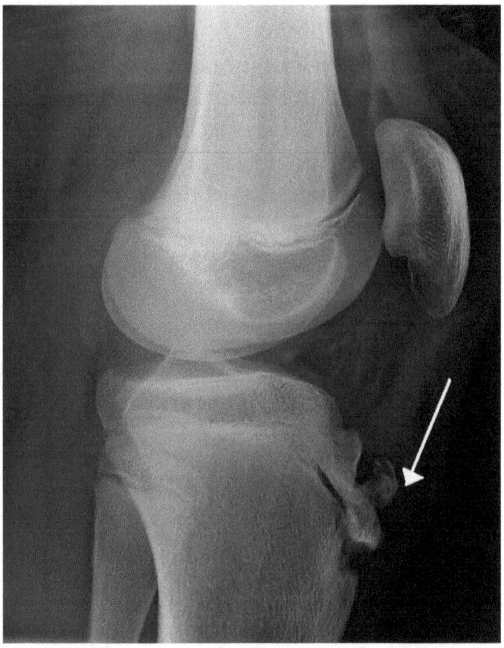

Ankle

The ankle consists of articulations among the three structures of the tibia, fibula, and talus. These three bones, along with the medial and lateral collateral ligaments and interosseous ligament, provide stability to the ankle joint (Figure 8.35). AP, lateral, and mortise views are necessary to fully evaluate the ankle. The AP view will demonstrate a longer lateral malleolus than the medial malleolus (Figure 8.36A). The mortise view requires an oblique view at 20° to 30° of internal rotation to allow for alignment of the lateral and medial malleoli (Figure 8.36B). Assess Bohler's angle by drawing one line tangent to the superior aspect of the calcaneus and the second line tangent to the inferior aspect of calcaneus. A normal Bohler's angle should be between 20° and 40°. The lateral view should show open collimation and include the calcaneus, base of the fifth metatarsal, and the dorsal surface of the talus and navicular bone (Figure 8.36C).

Trauma to the ankle can result from either inversion or eversion injury, direct blow, extreme dorsiflexion or plantar flexion, or a combination of all of these. Ligamentous damage can occur with or without an effusion, and most commonly occur from inversion causing soft tissue swelling of the lateral aspect of the ankle that may be visualized on the radiograph without an accompanied fracture. Joint

FIGURE 8.34 Osgood-Schlatter disease.
Source: Reprinted by permission of James Heilman, MD, Wikipedian, ER Deparment Head, East Kootenay Regional Hospital, Clinical Assistant Professor, Department of Emergency Medicine, University of British Columbia.

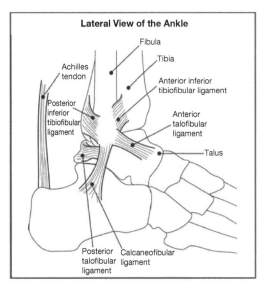

FIGURE 8.35 Ankle anatomy.
Source: https://en.wikipedia.org/wiki/Ankle

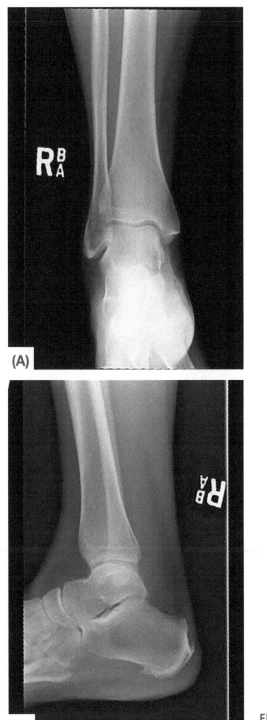

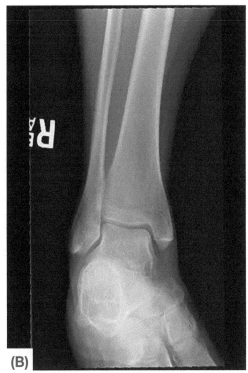

FIGURE 8.36 (A–C) Normal ankle x-ray views.
Source: Courtesy of Dr. David Begleiter.

effusions are most often seen in the anterior aspect of the ankle where fluid accumulates, appearing as a semicircular density anterior to the talotibial joint on the lateral view (**Figure 8.37**).

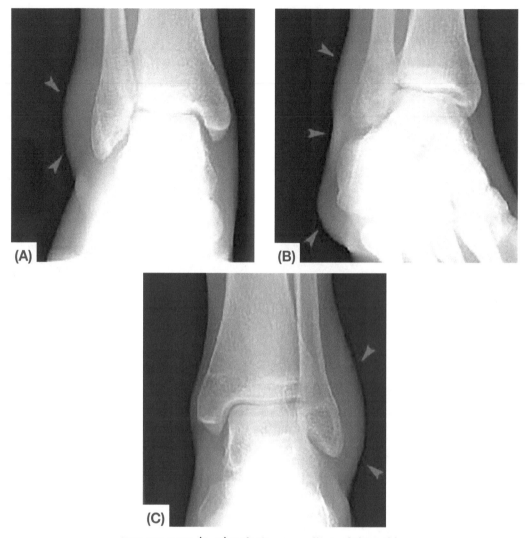

FIGURE 8.37 (A–C) Soft tissue swelling of the ankle.
Source: University of Virginia. Permission granted by the University of Virginia Department of
Radiology and Medical Imaging.

Mortise fractures can involve one, two, or all three of the bones that comprise the ankle. Since the ankle bones form a ring, if you identify a displaced fracture, carefully evaluate for another fracture. Ligamentous injuries of the medial collateral and lateral collateral ligaments may also rupture. If rupture occurs, there may be an accompanying avulsion fracture as well as soft tissue swelling. Ligamentous rupture can be assessed by scanning the radiograph approximately 1 cm proximal to the tibial plafond distribution found between the tibia and fibula. This area should not measure more than 6 mm (Figure 8.38).

When assessing for ankle fractures, scan the medial, lateral, and posterior malleolus and talus for any disruption, avulsion, or displacement. If an isolated distal fibula fracture or lateral malleolus fracture is identified, focus on the posterior aspect scanning for an accompanying fracture. If the medial malleolus or posterior malleolus shows a fracture with displacement, obtain a full-length tibia/fibula radiograph to assess for an

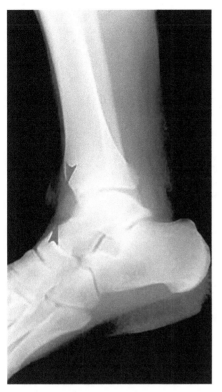

accompanying fracture. Look for widening of the medial joint space.

Accessory ossicles are unfused secondary ossification centers within the ankle. These ossicles will appear well corticated on imaging. An os subfibulare can be seen distal to the tip of the lateral malleolus. An os subtibiale can be seen distal to the tip of the medial malleolus. Theos trigonum is located posterior to the talus (Figure 8.39).

Foot

The foot is divided into three regions: the forefoot, midfoot, and hindfoot. The hindfoot consists of the talus and calcaneus. The midfoot includes the navicular, cuboid, and three cuneiforms. The metatarsals and phalanges make up the forefoot. When imaging the foot, obtaining AP, lateral, and oblique views (Figure 8.40). A tangential film aids in identifying abnormalities in the three regions of the foot. Fractures occur more often than dislocations. However, fractures and dislocations can occur simultaneously.

FIGURE 8.38 Ankle effusion.
Source: University of Virginia. Permission granted by the University of Virginia Department of Radiology and Medical Imaging.

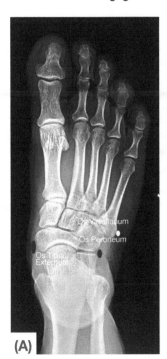

(A)

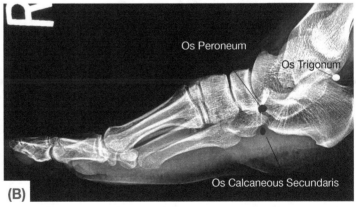

(B)

FIGURE 8.39 (A, B) Unfused secondary ossification centers.
Source: Courtesy of Dr. David Begleiter; diagramming by Theresa M. Campo.

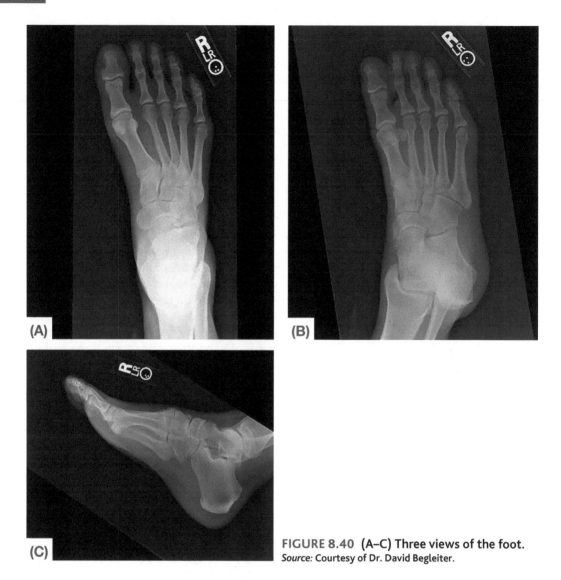

FIGURE 8.40 (A–C) Three views of the foot.
Source: Courtesy of Dr. David Begleiter.

Talus

The body of the talus includes the talar dome, which is divided into the medial and lateral aspects **(Figure 8.41)**. Fractures to the body of the talus often involve the medial and lateral aspects of the talar dome. Fractures to the talar neck can place a person at high risk for developing avascular necrosis. Inversion injuries of the ankle can cause avulsion fractures of the talus.

A talo-calcaneal coalition is defined as a union of one or more bones that are not normally fused. This is very rare and is not caused by a traumatic injury. Patients will complain of deep foot pain that is aggravated by activity, improves with rest, and appears as a partial or complete closure of the subtalar joint **(Figure 8.42)**.

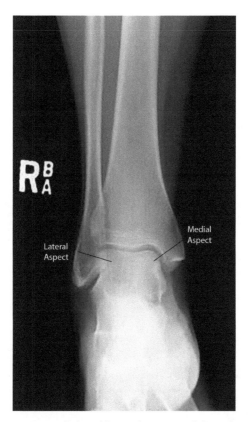

FIGURE 8.41 Medial and lateral aspect of the talar dome.
Source: Courtesy of Dr. David Begleiter; diagramming by Theresa M. Campo.

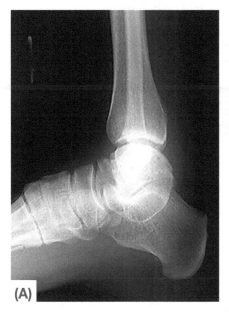

(A)

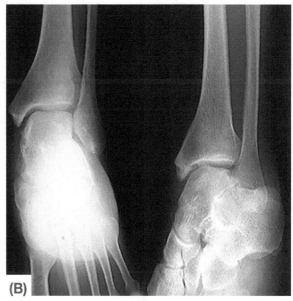

(B)

FIGURE 8.42 (A, B) Talo-calcaneal coalition.
Source: University of Virginia. Permission granted by the University of Virginia Department of Radiology and Medical Imaging.

Calcaneus

Calcaneal fractures most commonly occur from a high velocity fall from heights. They are identified by a Bohler's angle that is less than 20°. Compression fractures cannot be excluded if the Bohler's angle is within normal limits. Because of the mechanism of injury, these fractures are commonly associated with spinal compression fractures, femoral neck fractures, and tibial plateau fractures. If a calcaneal fracture or fractures are identified, order imaging of the hips and spine. Evaluation of the subtalar joint is also necessary when evaluating for calcaneal fractures on imaging. Stress fractures of the calcaneus can also occur and are mostly seen in runners and older adults. **Figure 8.43** demonstrates various calcaneal fractures found on radiograph.

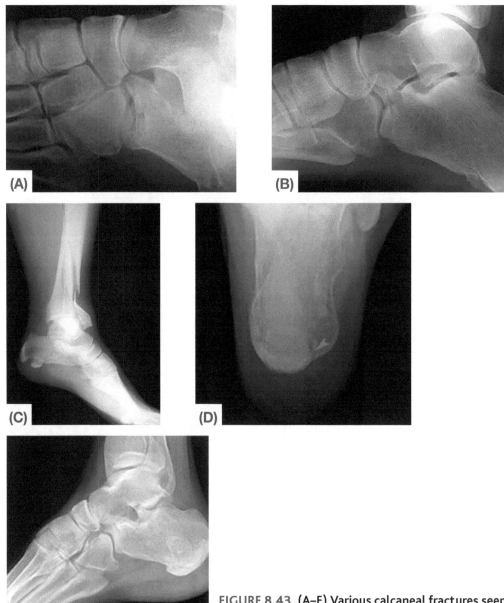

FIGURE 8.43 (A–E) Various calcaneal fractures seen on a radiograph.
Source: University of Virginia. Permission granted by the University of Virginia Department of Radiology and Medical Imaging.

Tarsals

The midfoot consists of the tarsal bones of the foot: the navicular, cuboid, and the three cunei-forms (Figure 8.44). Fractures can occur in any of these bones and should be evaluated on all images (Figure 8.45).

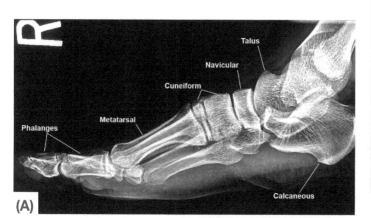
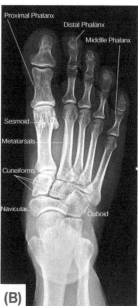

FIGURE 8.44 (A, B) Bones of the foot.
Source: Courtesy of Dr. Keith Lafferty; diagramming by Theresa M. Campo.

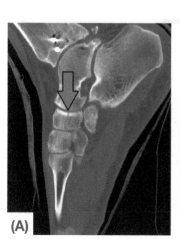
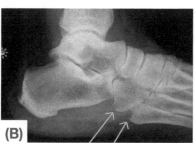
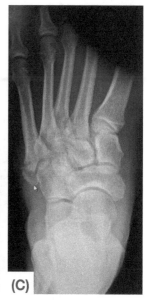

FIGURE 8.45 (A–C) Fractures of the tarsal bones.
Source: Reprinted by permission of James Heilman, MD, Wikipedian, ER Department Head, East Kootenay Regional Hospital, Clinical Assistant Professor, Department of Emergency Medicine, University of British Columbia.

Metatarsals

The five metatarsals are part of the forefoot. A fracture at the base of the fifth metatarsal that is at least 1.5 cm distal to the metatarsal styloid is known as a Jones fracture (Figure 8.46). Jones fractures are commonly confused with unfused apophysis and avulsion fractures of the metatarsal tuberosity at the insertion of the peroneus brevis tendon. A Jones fracture is not an avulsion injury. An unfused apophysis of the fifth metatarsal usually occurs in a lengthwise pattern and lies parallel to the long axis of the metatarsal (Figure 8.47). An avulsion fracture usually occurs from an inversion injury (running in heels), occurs at the metatarsal tuberosity at the insertion of the peroneus brevis tendon, or occurs from violent contraction with force.

A Lisfranc injury is a fracture with or without dislocation at the tarsometatarsal joint. This fracture may occur when riding a motorbike or mountain bike and getting the foot caught in the pedal clips or when jamming the foot from a fall down stairs. This fracture is named after Napoleon's surgeon who saw this type of injury from soldiers being knocked off horses with their foot still in the stirrup. The mechanism causes a traumatic dorsiflexion that may also involve rotation. Although an uncommon injury, it is important to consider in traumatic foot injuries. A Lisfranc injury will cause loss of normal alignment at the base of the second metatarsal. There may also be a fracture at the base of the second metatarsal with loss of alignment at the third metatarsal (Figure 8.48).

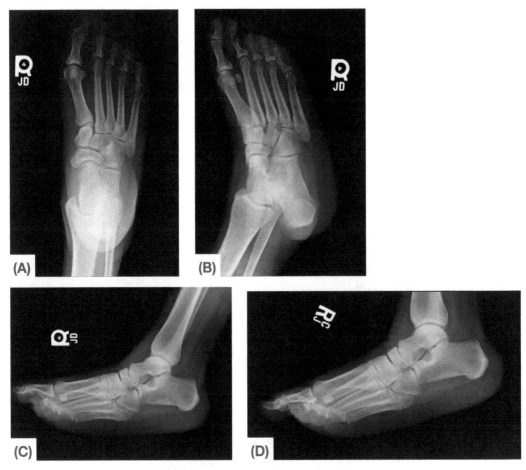

FIGURE 8.46 (A–D) Jones fracture.
Source: Courtesy of Dr. Douglas W. Parrillo.

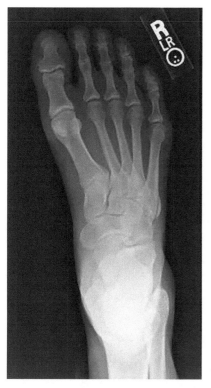

FIGURE 8.47 Unfused apophysis.
Source: Courtesy of Theresa M. Campo.

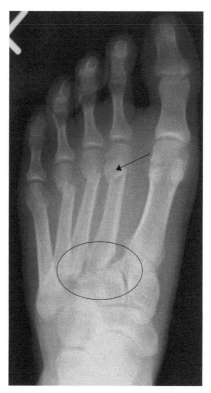

FIGURE 8.48 Lisfranc injury.
Source: Reprinted by permission of James Heilman, MD, Wikipedian, ER Department Head, East Kootenay Regional Hospital, Clinical Assistant Professor, Department of Emergency Medicine, University of British Columbia.

Midshaft fractures of the metatarsals may occur in one or in multiple metatarsals in a transverse oblique manner. Note if there is displacement and angulation, which affect treatment **(Figure 8.49)**.

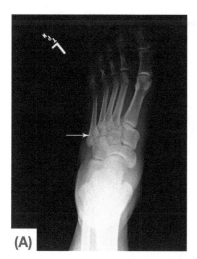

(A)

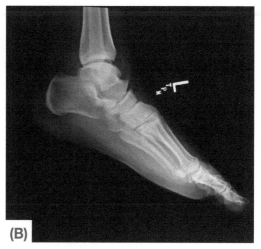

(B)

FIGURE 8.49 (A, B) Metatarsal fractures.
Source: Courtesy of Dr. Douglas W. Parrillo.

Phalanges

The phalanges make up the other part of the forefoot. Fractures most commonly occur in the proximal phalanx and may occur in one phalanx or multiple phalanges. Dislocations are also common in the toes and may be accompanied by fractures (Figure 8.50).

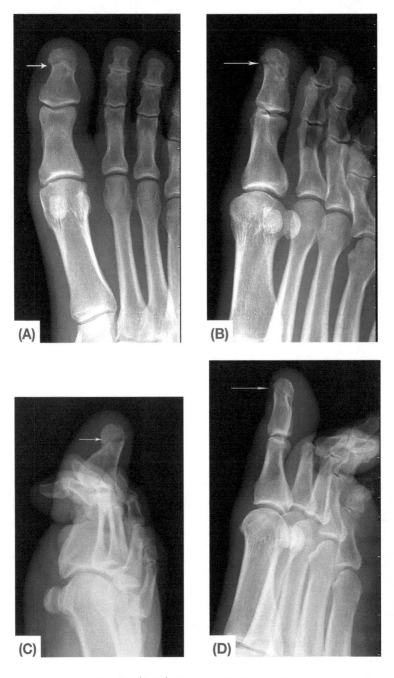

FIGURE 8.50 (A–D) First distal phalanx fractures.
Source: Courtesy of Kyle Deuter; diagramming by Theresa M. Campo.

CONCLUSION

The lower extremity consists of weight-bearing bones and complex joints along with soft tissues, including cartilage, ligaments, bursa, and muscle. These structures and inflammatory effusions can create challenges in identifying abnormalities.

RESOURCES

Au-Yong, I., Au-Yong, A., & Broderick, N. (2010). *On-call x-rays made easy*. Churchill Livingstone, Elsevier.

Daffner, R. H. (2014). Musculoskeletal imaging. In R. H. Daffner & M. S. Hartman (Eds.), *Clinical radiology: The essentials* (4th ed., pp. 353–429). Wolters Kluwer/Lippincott Williams & Wilkins.

Gray, H. (1918). *Anatomy of the human body*. Henry Vandyke Cater (illustrator). Lea and Febiger Publishers. https://en.wikipedia.org/wiki/Pelvis#/media/File:Gray241.png

McKinnis, L. N. (2020). *Fundamentals of musculoskeletal imaging* (5th ed.). F. A. Davis.

Helms, C. A. (2018). Miscellaneous bone lesions. In W. E. Brant & C. A. Helms (Eds.), *Fundamentals of diagnostic radiology* (5th ed., pp. 1090–1097). Wolters Kluwer/Lippincott Williams & Wilkins.

Helms, C. A. (2018). Skeletal trauma. In W. E. Brant & C. A. Helms (Eds.), *Fundamentals of diagnostic radiology* (5th ed., pp. 1015–1042). Wolters Kluwer/Lippincott Williams & Wilkins.

Herring, W. (2016). *Learning radiology: Recognizing the basics* (3rd ed., pp. 240–253). Elsevier.

Kuntz, A. F., Lai, W. S., Norton, P. T., Yao, L. L., & Gay, S. B. (n.d.). *Skeletal trauma*. https://introductiontoradiology.net/courses/rad/ext/

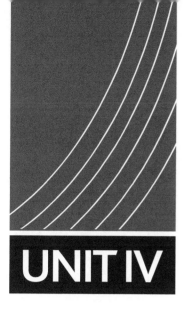

UNIT IV

Interpretation of Spine Radiographs

CHAPTER 9

Basic Interpretation of Cervical Spine Radiographs

► **VIDEO**

9.1: Interpretation—Normal Cervical Spine

Accompanying videos can be accessed online at https://connect.springerpub
.com/content/book/978-0-8261-6047-8/chapter/ch09

There are approximately 17,000 spinal injuries in the United States annually with the majority being males between 16 and 30 years of age (Ramirez & Campo, 2021). Historically, the standard for evaluating the spine has been radiographs. However, current data support the use of CT scanning for rapid evaluation of cervical spine injuries when available since 20% of cervical fractures are missed on radiographs.

Cervical spine imaging and interpretation of spinal radiographs can be challenging. Guidelines such as the National Emergency X-Radiography Utilization Study (NEXUS) criteria and the Canadian C-Spine (cervical spine) Rules (CCR) provide evidence-based guidelines for determining whether medical imaging is necessary. The NEXUS criteria are based on five factors: focal neural deficit, presence of midline spine tenderness, altered level of consciousness, presence of intoxication, and a distracting injury. The CCR has three categories with an algorithmic approach to decision-making for imaging:

1. If patient has any high-risk factors such as age older than 65 years, having a dangerous mechanism of injury, and/or presence of paresthesia, then spinal images are indicated.
2. If the patient does not have any of these risk factors but has pain with examination of the cervical spine and gentle passive range of motion, then imaging is warranted.
3. If no pain is elicited during the assessment, the patient is asked to actively rotate the neck; if any pain or limitation is noted, imaging is indicated.

Typically, three views of the cervical spine radiographic study are obtained. These include the anterior–posterior (AP), lateral, and odontoid views (Figure 9.1). The lateral view is performed first before spinal immobilization is removed. An adequate lateral view must include all seven vertebrae from C1 to the top of T1, including the junction of C7–T1 (Figure 9.2). If the patient has a thick neck or if soft tissue hinders the adequacy of the view, then traction on the arms, pulling downward toward the feet, can be performed to enhance the view. If this maneuver fails to improve the adequacy of the view, then a swimmer's view may be obtained. In a swimmer's view, the patient places one arm over their head, which aids in viewing the entire cervical spine. Once an adequate lateral image is obtained and visualized and no abnormalities are identified, the view should be repeated after the cervical collar is removed. In the AP view, the patient's mouth is closed during imaging, whereas in the odontoid view the mouth is kept open, which provides the best image of C1 and C2 (Figure 9.3).

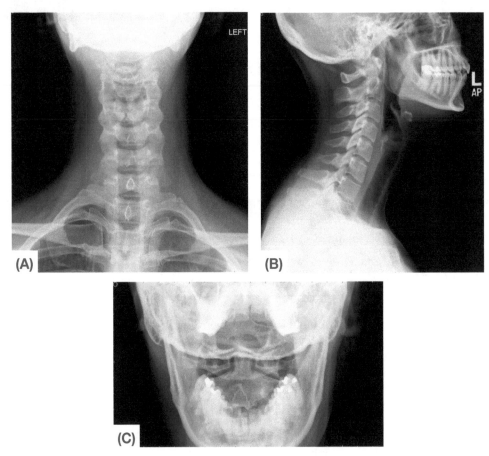

FIGURE 9.1 (A) Anterior–posterior view; (B) lateral view; (C) odontoid view.
Source: Courtesy of Theresa M. Campo.

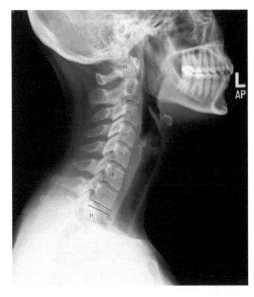

FIGURE 9.2 Normal lateral view including T1 and showing the C7–T1 junction.
Source: Courtesy of Theresa M. Campo.

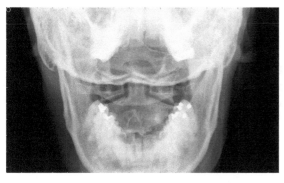

FIGURE 9.3 **Odontoid view.**
Note: The mouth is open allowing for visualization of C1 and C2.
Source: Courtesy of Theresa M. Campo.

If pain is present and there are no signs of any abnormalities with the routine three views, then a flexion and extension view can be obtained (Figure 9.4). A CT scan is not mandatory for evaluating the cervical spine, but if there are any injuries questioned or suspected on plain radiographs then it should be considered. CT scanning may also be considered in the older adult patient to improve identification of fractures which may be difficult to appreciate with arthritic changes on plain films. If ligamentous injury, neurological deficits, or spinal canal involvement are either suspected or confirmed by plain radiographs, a CT scan or MRI of the cervical spine should be obtained since they are excellent at contrasting soft tissue.

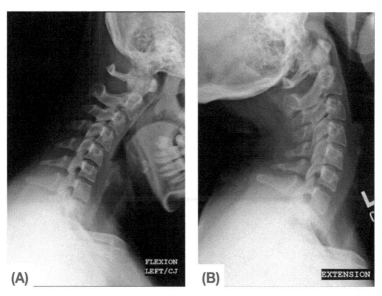

(A)   FLEXION LEFT/CJ   (B)   EXTENSION

FIGURE 9.4 **(A) Flexion view; (B) extension view.**
Source: Courtesy of Dr. Douglas W. Parrillo.

NORMAL

When evaluating the cervical spine on plain radiographs, it is important to look at each view in its entirety; however, your approach may be slightly different from one image to the other with regard to the ABCDs that we have been using throughout this text. We will talk about each view in detail with regard to visualizing normal and identifying abnormal findings.

Lateral View

The lateral view is best for detecting most abnormalities in cervical spine radiographs. Before beginning interpretation of the lateral view, it is important to ensure *a*dequacy. The provider must be able to visualize from C1 down to at least the top of T1, including the C7–T1 junction (see **Figure 9.2**). It is also important to identify that there is good penetration with contrast occurring between the bony structures and the soft tissue.

A—When assessing for *a*lignment, there are four anatomical lines that need to be evaluated. The first two lines should be drawn from the odontoid peg through to the top of T1 along the anterior margin and posterior margin of the vertebral bodies. The third line should be drawn along the spinolaminar junction and a fourth line should be along the posterior spinous processes. See **Figure 9.5** to view all four lines. The spinolaminar (posterior margin of the spinal canal) line may have a slight step at C2 posteriorly in children but should not exceed 2 mm. All the lines should follow the normal cervical lordotic curve with no breaks in the lines or stair stepping (step-off), which may be indicative of a ligamentous injury or occult fracture. There may be straightening of the cervical lordotic curve that can be normal or from muscle spasm.

B—Next, the *b*one structures need to be evaluated in detail. Each vertebra from C2 downward should be rectangular in shape and similar in size with the anterior aspect being of similar height to the posterior aspect. If the anterior aspect is greater than 3 mm narrower than the posterior aspect, then a wedge fracture should be suspected. The normal bone structures of the cervical spine are outlined in **Figure 9.6**. Note the pedicles, facet joint, lamina, spinous process, and lateral mass.

C—The *c*artilaginous spaces are evaluated next. The area between the dens, a projection of the axis of C2, and the body of C1 is known as the predental space and should not measure more than 3 mm in an adult or 5 mm in children (**Figure 9.7**). If the predental space is greater than specified, then a fracture to the odontoid process or disruption of the transverse ligament should be suspected. If either is suspected, further imaging with either CT or MRI should be performed.

D—The *d*isc spaces should be similar anteriorly and posteriorly between each vertebra and similar in height along the cervical spine. Decreases in disc space may occur from

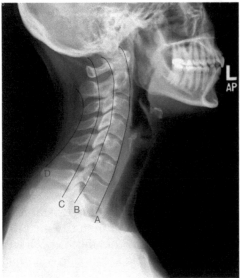

FIGURE 9.5 **Four anatomical lines.**
Note: A, anterior vertebral; B, posterior vertebral; C, spinolaminar; D, posterior spinous process.
Source: Courtesy of Theresa M. Campo.

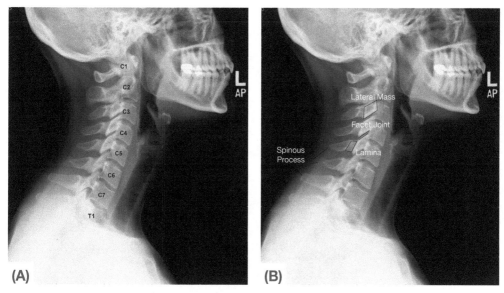

(A)   **(B)**

FIGURE 9.6 **(A) Cervical vertebrae C1 through the top of T1. Note the shape and alignment of each vertebra. (B) Normal cervical bone structures. Note the lateral mass, facet joint, lamina, and spinous process in addition to the vertebral bodies.**
Source: Courtesy of Theresa M. Campo.

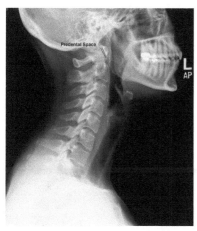

FIGURE 9.7 **Predental space.**
Source: Courtesy of Theresa M. Campo.

degenerative changes. However, if a decrease in height is noted, an MRI should be considered to evaluate the possibility of a disc herniation.

The nasopharyngeal, retropharyngeal, and retrotracheal space should be evaluated for soft tissue swelling **(Figure 9.8)**. The nasopharyngeal space anterior to C1 should not measure more than 10 mm. The retropharyngeal space anterior to C2 to C3/C4 should measure between 4 mm and 7 mm and the retrotracheal space anterior to C5 to C7 should not exceed 14 mm in children and 22 mm in adults. Increased measurements in these areas may be indicative of a vertebral fracture causing bleeding or hematoma formation and require further imaging.

The AP view is often overlooked but valuable in identifying some fractures better than are seen on the lateral view. After determining *a*dequacy, *a*lignment should be evaluated

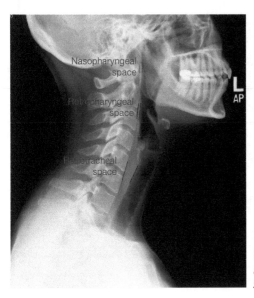

FIGURE 9.8 **Nasopharyngeal, retropharyngeal, and retrotracheal spaces.**
Source: Courtesy of Theresa M. Campo.

by looking at vertebral body edges and the articular pillars. The spinal processes should be midline and aligned in the vertical plane. If malalignment is identified, and the patient's head is not turned or shifted, a facet joint dislocation should be suspected. Each cervical vertebral body height and the intervertebral joint spaces should also be equal. The distance between the spinous processes in the vertical plane should also be equal. If the space between the spinous processes exceeds more than half the width of the vertebral body above or below, suspect an anterior cervical dislocation. See **Figure 9.9** for a normal AP view with markings.

The odontoid view is considered adequate if it allows for visualization of C1 and C2, including the entire odontoid and lateral borders of C1. Alignment of the occipital condyle with the lateral mass and superior articular facet of C1 should be visualized. The lateral

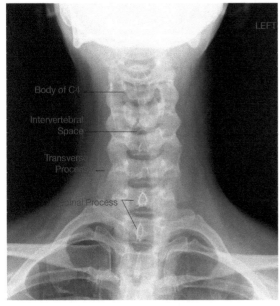

FIGURE 9.9 **Anterior–posterior view with markings.**
Source: Courtesy of Theresa M. Campo.

masses of C1 should not overhang the lateral masses of C2. There should be symmetry of the space between the dens in the lateral masses bilaterally of C1. See **Figure 9.10** for a normal odontoid view with markings. If the spaces are asymmetrical, evaluate the film to see if the patient has their head tilted to one side. If the head does not appear to be tilted to one side, then joint space asymmetry may be suggestive of a C1 or C2 fracture. The odontoid should blend with the body of C2 and should not have any disruptions of the cortical margins. If there is disruption of the cortical margins, then a fracture should be suspected.

Soft tissue, tooth shadows, or the occiput can produce shadows that may mimic a fracture. To avoid this mistake, outline the shadow that is going through the odontoid to see if it progresses past the cortical margins of the odontoid itself. If you can discern an absolute outline of an underlying or overlapping structure, no further imaging is necessary. However, if you are not able to do this or if there is any question whatsoever, further imaging should be obtained.

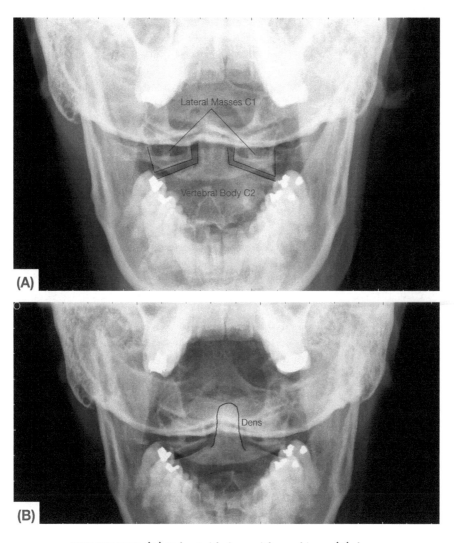

FIGURE 9.10 (A) Odontoid view with markings; (B) dens.
Source: Courtesy of Theresa M. Campo.

If pain persists and no abnormalities are identified on the three routine views, additional views such as oblique as well as flexion and extension can be considered. Oblique views are taken at a 45° angle and can increase visibility of the intervertebral foramina in the presence of spondylosis of the facet joints. The right posterior oblique demonstrates the left foramina and the right anterior oblique demonstrates the right foramina.

Flexion and extension views are used to visualize ligament instability and to assess vertebral mobility. If mild malalignment is identified on routine views, the flexion and extension is especially useful in the trauma patient to rule out ligamentous injury when there is minimal malalignment seen on plain radiographs.

Cervical spine trauma is most often seen with the cervical spine in hyperflexion. This is because when the head is flexed the force exerts itself on the C4 through C7 vertebral bodies, causing compression of the vertebral bodies and anterior wedging. In the posterior aspect, the lamina within the spinal processes and the supporting ligaments are placed in tension, resulting in fracture and tears. Hyperextension injuries are less common, occurring only 20% of the time. These injuries result from tension on the anterior longitudinal ligament which may tear at the margin of the vertebral body or the intervertebral disc space. Hyperextension injuries can include avulsion fractures when the vertebral body is affected, fracture of the spinal processes posteriorly, and fracture of the lamina and facets. Axial trauma can cause compression to the intervertebral disc causing comminuted vertebral body fractures.

If the patient has a distraction injury, assessment for head trauma or spinal injury is necessary. Distraction injuries include extremity fractures or severe sprains, as well as chest, abdominal, or back trauma. Rotation injuries can cause fractures in the posterior elements of the spine, especially the facets and lamina, and result in fracture dislocation. Always maintain stability of the cervical spine if injury is strongly suspected by using cervical immobilization devices such as a cervical collar, cervical immobilization device (CID), or equivalent equipment.

ABNORMALITIES

Abnormalities can occur anywhere along the cervical spine and involve either bone fractures or ligamentous injury. Using the NEXUS or CCR can assist in determining whether spinal imaging is warranted in identifying abnormalities. Any injury to the upper cervical area can be life-threatening and must be identified as soon as possible. Most cervical fractures occur between C3 and C7.

A Jefferson fracture occurs from compression of the bony ring of the C1 vertebra (Figure 9.11). This is caused by an axial load to the vertex of the head, usually from a diving injury. The fracture involves the anterior and posterior arches of C1 bilaterally with displacement of the C1 lateral masses beyond the margin of the body of C2. If lateral displacement is more than 2 mm or if unilateral displacement occurs, a C1 fracture may be present. If this is suspected, a CT scan is required to identify and delineate the extent of the fracture and possible impingement. Jefferson fractures are considered unstable and must be addressed immediately to avoid devastating neurological and life-threatening sequelae.

Fractures to the odontoid are best seen on the lateral view and are suspected with an anterior tilt or movement of the odontoid. This may be the only sign of a fracture and may be accompanied by prevertebral soft tissue swelling. Odontoid fractures are divided into three types. Type I is a fracture of the superior tip of the odontoid. It is relatively rare and can potentially be unstable. Type II odontoid fractures occur at the base of the odontoid, are the most common type, and are considered unstable. Type III odontoid fractures occur through the base of the odontoid into the body of the axis and have the best prognosis. See Figures 9.12, 9.13, and 9.14 for the three types of odontoid fractures.

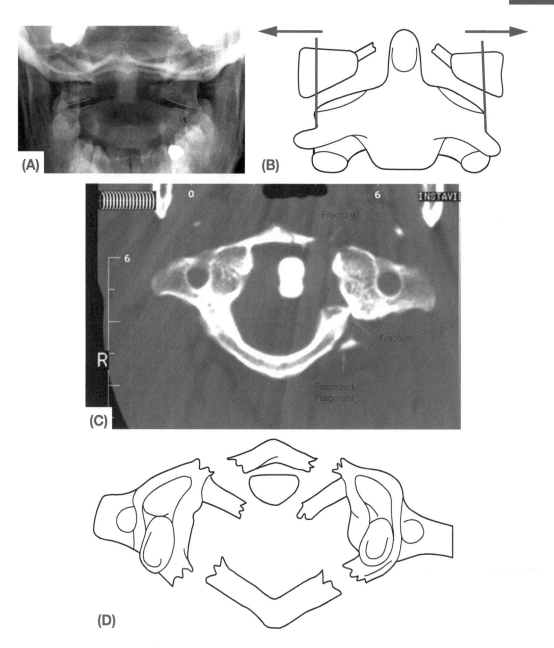

FIGURE 9.11 (A) Jefferson fracture on radiograph; (B) drawing depicting the injury;
(C) the fracture on CT scan slice; (D) drawing depicting the injury.
Source: University of Virginia. Permission granted by the University of
Virginia Department of Radiology and Medical Imaging.

A fracture through the pars interarticularis of the axis of C2 is known as a hangman's fracture (Figure 9.15). This fracture occurs from hyperextension such as in a motor vehicle accident when the head hits the dashboard. This fracture is accompanied by prevertebral soft tissue swelling and avulsion of the anterior inferior corner of C2. Additionally, there may be rupture of the anterior longitudinal ligament, anterior dislocation of the C2 vertebral body, and bilateral pars interarticularis fractures. A hangman's fracture is considered unstable and is best seen on the lateral view.

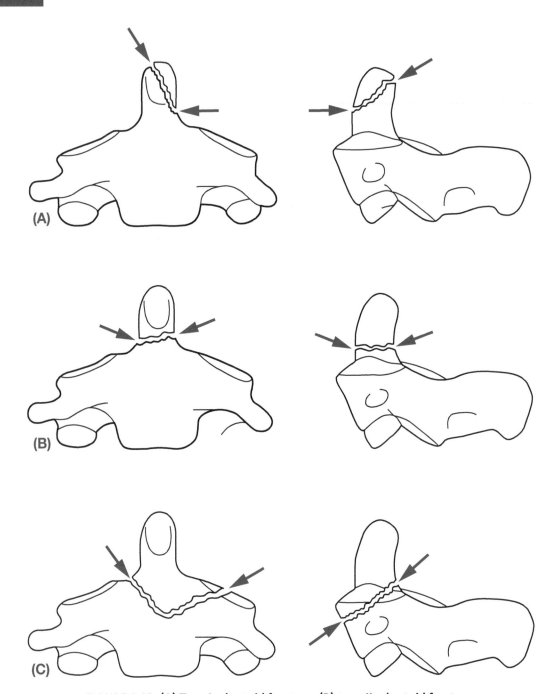

FIGURE 9.12 (A) Type I odontoid fracture; (B) type II odontoid fracture;
(C) type III odontoid fracture.
Source: University of Virginia. Permission granted by the University of
Virginia Department of Radiology and Medical Imaging.

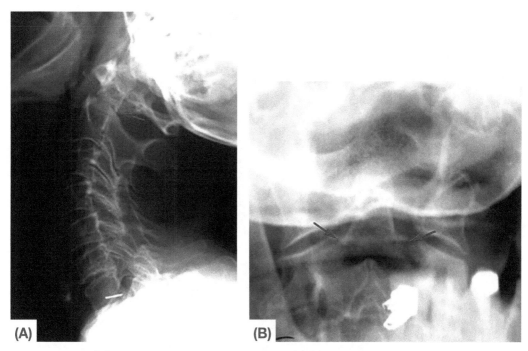

FIGURE 9.13 (A) Type II dens fracture lateral view; (B) type II dens fracture odontoid view.
Source: University of Virginia. Permission granted by the University of Virginia Department of Radiology and Medical Imaging.

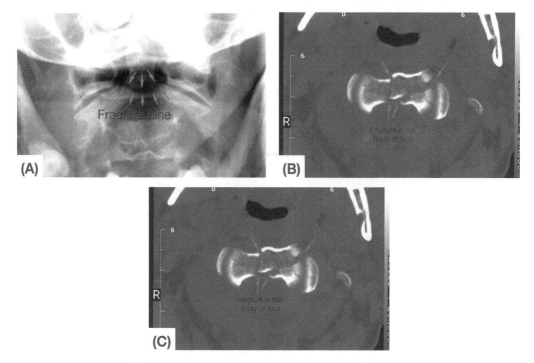

FIGURE 9.14 (A) Type III dens fracture odontoid view; (B) type III dens fracture; (C) type III dens fracture. Note clarity with CT image.
Source: University of Virginia. Permission granted by the University of Virginia Department of Radiology and Medical Imaging.

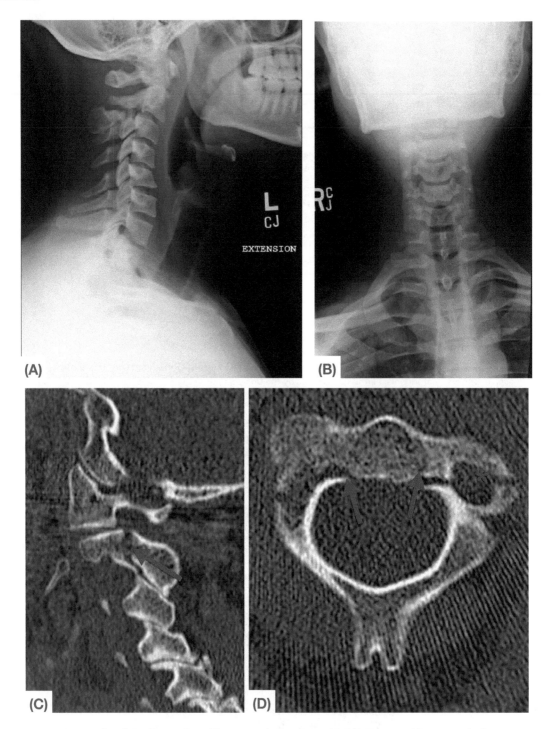

FIGURE 9.15 (A,B) Radiographs of hangman's fracture; (C,D)CT scan of hangman's fracture.
Source: (A,B) Courtesy of Dr. Douglas W. Parrillo; (C,D) courtesy of Utz, M., Khan, S., O'Connor, D., & Meyers, S. (2013). MDCT and MRI evaluation of cervical spine trauma. *Insights into Imaging, 5*(1), 67–75. https://doi .org/10.1007/s13244-013-0304-2

A teardrop fracture occurs when there is an anterior compression fracture of the vertebral body resulting from a severe flexion injury, such as diving into shallow water (Figure 9.16). There may also be posterior ligament disruption as well as prevertebral swelling associated with the anterior longitudinal ligament tear. This avulsion fracture resembles a teardrop on the lateral view. There may also be posterior vertebral body subluxation into the spinal canal with spinal cord compression and instability. This injury may also be accompanied by a fracture of the spinous process as well as vertebral body displacement and is considered unstable.

Complete anterior dislocation of the vertebral body resulting from extreme flexion of the head and neck without axial compression results in bilateral facet dislocation, is considered unstable, and is associated with a high risk for spinal cord damage. There may be complete anterior dislocation of the vertebral body by half its AP diameter. Disruption of the posterior and anterior longitudinal ligament may accompany this injury, causing a bowtie or batwing appearance of the locked facets. This injury is best seen on the lateral view (Figure 9.17).

In contrast, a unilateral facet dislocation and rupture of the apophyseal joint ligaments can result from an anterior dislocation of the affected vertebral body by less than half of the vertebral body AP diameter. There may also be discordant rotation above and below the involved level best seen as a widening of the disc space on the oblique. Again, a bowtie or batwing appearance of the overriding locked facet within the intervertebral foramina may occur. This injury is considered stable and results from flexion and rotation occurring simultaneously. See Figure 9.18 showing a unilateral facet dislocation.

Anterior subluxation occurs when there is disruption of the posterior ligamentous complex with loss of normal cervical lordosis and anterior displacement of the vertebral body accompanied by fanning of the interspinous distance. This is considered to be unstable if the anterior subluxation is more than 4 mm with an associated compression fracture of more than 20% of the affected vertebral body height, with an increase or decrease in normal disc space, and if fanning occurs of the interspinous distance. This may be difficult to diagnose if muscle spasms present simultaneously. This injury may be stable initially

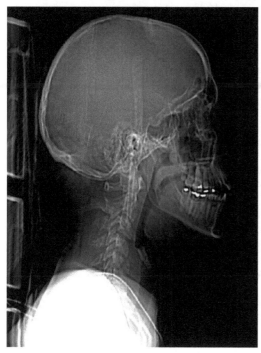

FIGURE 9.16 **Teardrop fracture.**
Source: Courtesy of Dr. Douglas W. Parrillo.

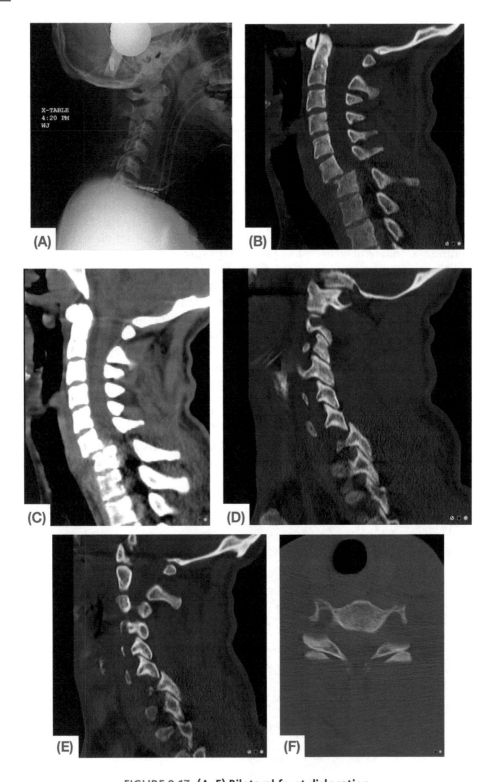

FIGURE 9.17 (A–F) Bilateral facet dislocation.
Source: (A) Courtesy of Dr. Douglas W. Parrillo. (B–F) with permission from Dr. Chris O'Donnell, Radiopaedia.org,
rID: 21424 (https://radiopaedia.org/articles/bilateral-facet-dislocation).

and then may become unstable 20% to 50% of the time with hyperflexion of the neck. See Figure 9.19 for anterior subluxation.

Clay shoveler's fracture is a fracture of the C6 to T1 spinal process. This injury is often caused by hyperflexion with contraction of the paraspinous muscles, which avulse the spinal process itself. This fracture is best viewed in the lateral view. It is considered stable and may be accompanied by a ghost sign on the AP view, caused by the overlapping of the spinal processes of C6 or C7 due to the displaced fracture. See Figure 9.20 for clay shoveler's fracture.

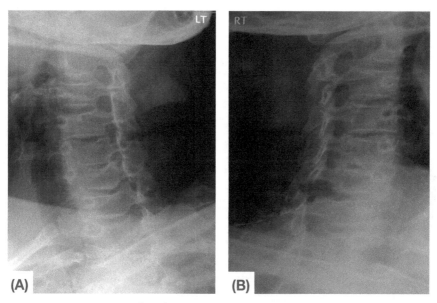

FIGURE 9.18 (A, B) Unilateral locked facet with fracture.
Source: Courtesy of Dr. Douglas W. Parrillo.

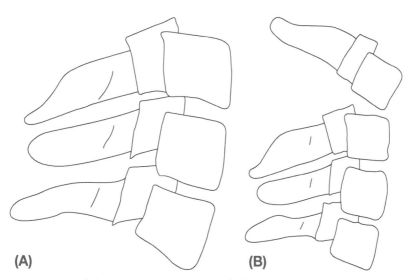

FIGURE 9.19 (A) Normal cervical spine; (B) anterior subluxation C spine.
Note the malalignment of the anterior line.
Source: Courtesy of Theresa M. Campo.

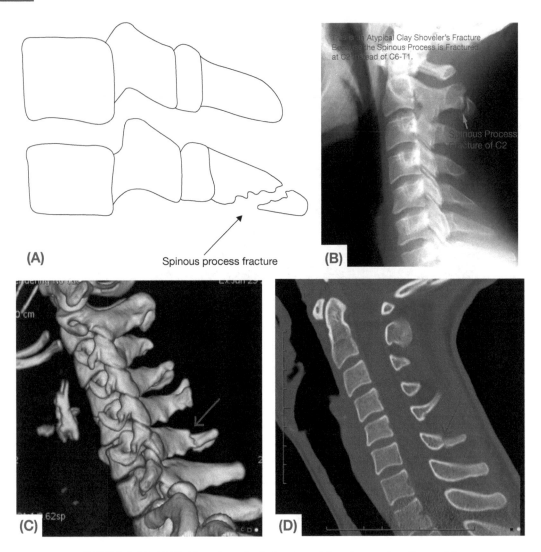

FIGURE 9.20 (A,B) Clay shoveler's fracture (drawing and radiograph); (C) 3D VR bone window; (D) sagittal bone view CT scan.
Source: (A,B) University of Virginia. Permission granted by the University of
Virginia Department of Radiology and Medical Imaging; (C,D) courtesy of Dr. Chris O'Donnell, Radiopaedia.org,
rID: 27426 (https://radiopaedia.org/cases/clay-shoveler-fracture-7).

A wedge fracture is a compression fracture caused by hyperflexion and compression that causes buckling of the anterior cortex and loss of height of the anterior vertebral body with anterior superior fracture of the vertebral body (**Figure 9.21**). Burst fractures can occur at the levels of C3 through C7 from axial compression (**Figure 9.22**). This injury can cause damage to the spinal cord from the displacement of the posterior fragments and requires CT for further evaluation, although it is considered a stable fracture.

Atlanto-occipital dislocation is the separation of the skull from the cervical spine. This injury commonly occurs when a person is ejected from a motor vehicle, especially children younger than 2 years of age (**Figure 9.23**).

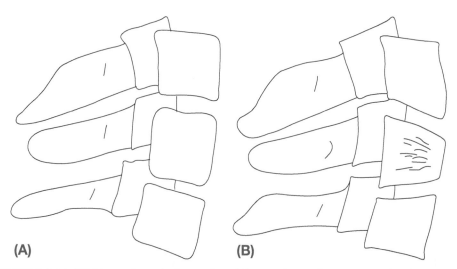

(A) **(B)**

FIGURE 9.21 **(A)** Normal cervical vertebra; **(B)** anterior wedge compression fracture.
Source: Courtesy of Theresa M. Campo.

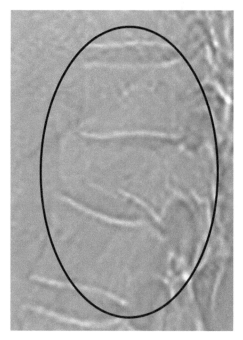

FIGURE 9.22 **Burst fracture.**
Source: Courtesy of Dr. Douglas W. Parrillo.

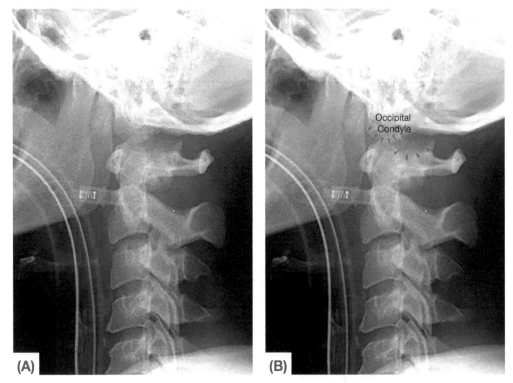

FIGURE 9.23 (A,B) Atlanto-occipital dislocation.
Note the anterior displacement of the occipital condyles.
Source: University of Virginia. Permission granted by the University of
Virginia Department of Radiology and Medical Imaging.

Osteoarthritic degenerative changes in the cervical spine occur with aging, including loss of disc height, bone spurring, and increased prevertebral space swelling. These changes make it challenging to evaluate acute injuries with plain radiograph images. Therefore, imaging for acute injury using CT or MRI may be necessary to evaluate the cervical bones and to assess the spinal cord for any abnormalities, including partial compression stenosis or complete nerve root impingement.

CONCLUSION

It is important to obtain adequate films along with careful assessment of neurological status to ensure accurate interpretation of cervical spine conditions. Cervical spine radiographs may be beneficial in identifying fractures, subluxations, dislocations, and degenerative changes. Closely adhering to evidence-based guidelines such as the NEXUS and CCR criteria will reduce the likelihood of inappropriate imaging. However, the provider should remember that degenerative changes and abnormalities noted with plain films may warrant imaging with CT or MRI to avoid missing potentially life-threatening or debilitating spinal cord trauma.

RESOURCES

American Association of Neurological Surgeons. (n.d.). *Spinal cord injury*. https://www .aans.org/Patients/Neurosurgical-Conditions-and-Treatments/Spinal-Cord-Injury

Auyeung, S., MacLeod, T. D., & Lazaro, R. T. (2020). Radiologic evaluation of the cervical spine. In L. N. McKinnis (Ed.), *Fundamentals of musculoskeletal imaging* (5th ed.). F. A. Davis.

Au-Yong, I., Au-Yong, A., & Broderick, N. (2010). *On-call x-rays made easy*. Churchill Livingstone, Elsevier.

Barakos, J. A., & Purcell, D. D. (2018). Head and neck imaging. In W. E. Brant & C. A. Helms (Eds.), *Fundamentals of diagnostic radiology* (5th ed., pp. 240–266). Wolters Kluwer/ Lippincott Williams & Wilkins.

Committee on Trauma. (2018). *ATLS Advanced Trauma Life Support student course manual* (10th ed.). American College of Surgeons.

Daffner, R. H. (2014). Musculoskeletal imaging. In R. H. Daffner & M. S. Hartman (Eds.), *Clinical radiology: The essentials* (4th ed., pp. 482–533). Wolters Kluwer/Lippincott Williams & Wilkins.

Davenport, M. (2017). *Cervical spine fracture evaluation*. Medscape. https://emedicine .medscape.com/article/824380-overview

Herring, W. (2016). *Learning radiology: Recognizing the basics* (3rd ed., pp. 266–278). Elsevier.

Nickson, C. (2019). *Cervical spine assessment*. https://litfl.com/cervical-spine-assessment

Ramirez, E. G., & Campo, T. M. (2021). Clearing the cervical spine. In T. M. Campo and K. A. Lafferty (Eds.): *Essential procedures for emergency, urgent, and primary care settings: A clinical companion* (3rd ed.). Springer Publishing Company.

Stiell, I. G., Clement, C. M., McKnight, R. D., Brison, R, Schull, M. J., Rowe, B. H., Worthington, J. R., Eisenhauer, M. A., Cass, D., Greenberg, G., MacPhail, I., Dreyer, J., Lee, J. S., Bandiera, G., Reardon, M., Holroyd, B., & Lesiuk, H. (2003). The Canadian C-spine rule versus the NEXUS—Low-risk criteria in patients with trauma. *New England Journal of Medicine, 349*, 2510–2518. https://doi.org/10.1056/NEJMoa031375

University of Virginia Department of Radiology and Medical Imaging. (n.d.). *Introduction to radiology*. https://www.med-ed.virginia.edu/courses/rad/

Utz, M., Khan, S., O'Connor, D., & Meyers, S. (2013). MDCT and MRI evaluation of cervical spine trauma. *Insights into Imaging, 5*(1), 67–75. https://doi.org/10.1007 /s13244-013-0304-2

Yao, L. L., Gay, S. B., Vu, Q. D. M., Anderson, M. W., Powell, S. M., & Patel, P. N. (n.d.). *Imaging evaluation of the cervical spine*. https://introductiontoradiology.net/courses /rad/cspine/

CHAPTER 10

Basic Interpretation of Thoracic Spine Radiographs

▶ VIDEO

10.1: Interpretation—Normal Thoracic and Lumbar Spine

Accompanying videos can be accessed online at https://connect.springerpub.com/content/book/978-0-8261-6047-8/chapter/ch10

Numerous conditions can predispose a person to a spinal injury, including degeneration, malignancy, loss of bone density, Paget's disease, autoimmune disorders, hemorrhagic disease, and congenital disorders or malformations. The thoracic spine is generally better protected than the cervical spine and greater forces are needed to cause serious injury. Because of this, injuries of the thoracic spine may be associated with additional injuries of the chest and abdomen, including rib fractures and abdominal organ injuries. Remember to protect the spine during assessment by maintaining alignment and stabilization and to treat life-threatening injuries first.

Thoracic spine injuries should be suspected in patients who present after a fall, have multiple injuries, have a neurological deficit, or have a mechanism of severe local force. Injuries should also be suspected in patients with fractures to the sternum, the ribs, or the scapula. In patients who are elderly or have osteoporosis, it does not take a great deal of force to cause a wedge or compression fracture in the thoracic spine. In fact, simply rolling over in bed may cause a compression fracture with severe osteoporosis. In general, most fractures of the thoracic spine occur in the lower two thirds.

NORMAL

Thoracic radiographs generally involve two views: the anterior–posterior (AP) view and the lateral view. Adequate films require that the lower cervical (top of C7) and upper lumbar spine (top of L2) are included on both views **(Figure 10.1)**. When evaluating the AP and lateral views, there should be symmetry in the height of each of the vertebrae and equal spacing between the vertebrae and spinal processes. However, it is important to note that the vertebral body and intervertebral disc spaces become slightly larger at the base of the thoracic spine at the junction with the lumbar spine (T12 and L1).

When evaluating the AP view, the pedicle, spinous process, and transverse processes should be easily visualized **(Figure 10.2)**. On the lateral view, one should visualize the vertebral bodies and pedicles **(Figure 10.3)**. When reviewing thoracic spine images, view the outline of each vertebral body, pedicle, and transverse and spinal process systematically. Evaluate the distance between the pedicles as well as the vertebral disc spaces. The vertebral bodies should have smooth margins from the base of the cervical spine through the top of the lumbar spine. Any disruptions in alignment and/or disc spaces may be indicative of injury.

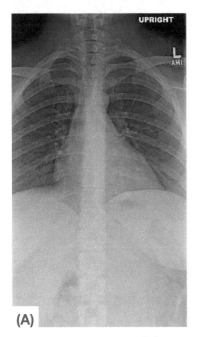

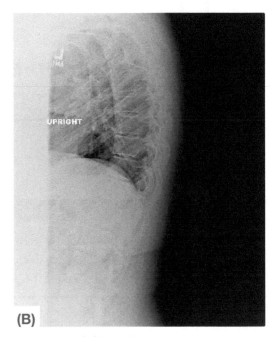

FIGURE 10.1 (A) Anterior–posterior view T spine; (B) lateral view T spine.
Source: Radiograph.

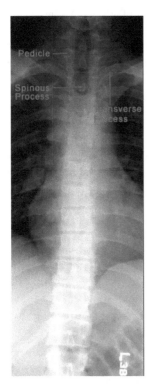

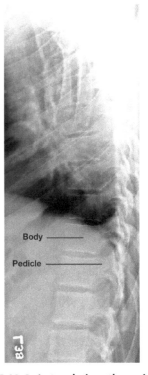

FIGURE 10.2 Anterior–posterior view thoracic spine with markings.
Source: University of Virginia. Permission granted by the University of Virginia Department of Radiology and Medical Imaging.

FIGURE 10.3 Lateral view thoracic spine with markings.
Source: University of Virginia. Permission granted by the University of Virginia Department of Radiology and Medical Imaging.

A—Image adequacy should be ensured prior to interpretation as with any other radiograph. Evaluating *a*lignment begins with the spinal processes. They should be readily visible on the AP view from the base of the cervical spine through to T4 or T5 and then again at the lower end of the thoracic spine. Both the anterior and posterior margins of the vertebra should be in alignment on the lateral view.

B—The vertebral *b*one (body) should have uniform margins that are aligned with no interruption in the margins. The pedicles should be visualized on the lateral view without any disruptions along their borders. It is important to note that in the lateral view the first four vertebral bodies are not readily visible because they are obscured by the shoulder girdle, superimposed ribs, and lung markings.

C—There is no *c* when interpreting the thoracic spine.

D—The intervertebral *d*isc spaces should get progressively larger with progression toward the lumbar spine.

S—The paravertebral *s*oft tissue line may be visible and is considered normal. However, any enhancement and/or displacement of this line suggests swelling and an injury. See **Figures 10.4 and 10.5** for interpretation of the thoracic spine.

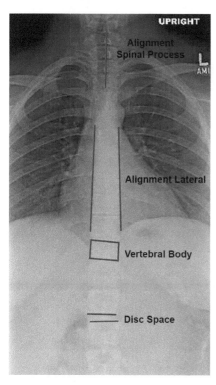

FIGURE 10.4 Anterior–posterior view interpretation.
Source: Courtesy of Dr. David Begleiter; diagramming by Theresa M. Campo.

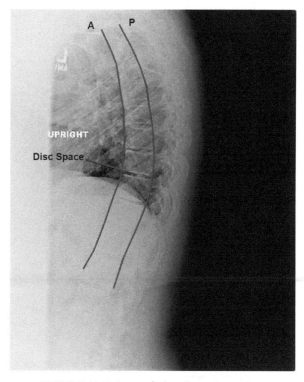

FIGURE 10.5 Lateral view interpretation.
Source: Courtesy of Dr. David Begleiter; diagramming by Theresa M. Campo.

ABNORMALITIES

There are three common mechanisms that cause injury to the thoracic spine: hyperflexion, vertical compression, and shearing injury. Hyperflexion, which causes anterior compression of the vertebral body known as wedging, is most common. See **Figure 10.6** demonstrating anterior compression or wedge fracture.

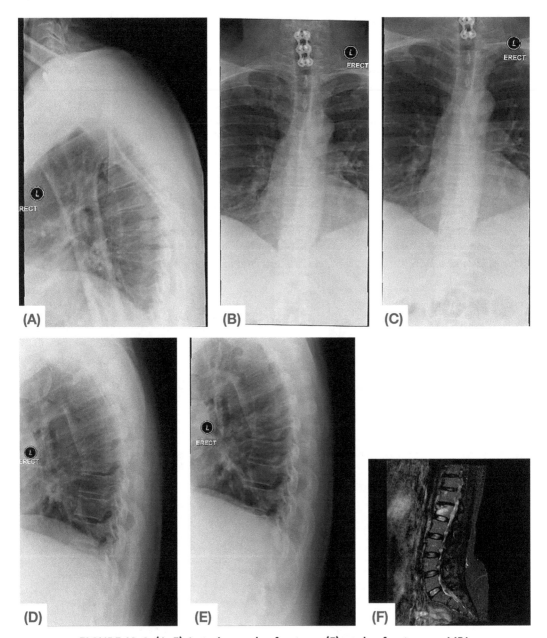

FIGURE 10.6 (A–E) Anterior wedge fracture; (F) wedge fracture on MRI.
Source: (A–E) Courtesy of Dr. David Parrillo; (F) courtesy of Dr. Dalia Ibrahim, Radiopaedia.org, rID: 28778
(https://radiopaedia.org/articles/spinal-wedge-fracture?lang=us).

Vertical compression can cause loss of height to the vertebral body in a crushing manner. See **Figure 10.7**, which demonstrates a compression fracture. The severity of the compression to the vertebra may vary. There is a natural tapering of the anterior thoracic vertebral body that should not be confused with a compression fracture which causes a loss of height along with disruption of the posterior line. Compression fractures are more common in women than men and may occur secondary to osteoporosis with minimal force.

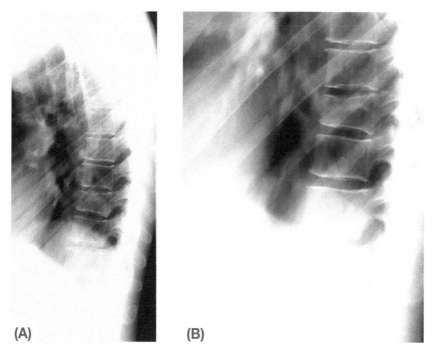

(A)   (B)

FIGURE 10.7 (A,B) Thoracic compression fracture.
Note compressed look to vertebra compared with surrounding vertebrae.
Source: University of Virginia. Permission granted by the University
of Virginia Department of Radiology and Medical Imaging.

A high-energy axial load can cause the disc above a vertebra to be driven downward, causing the vertebra to burst. This may cause fragments to be pushed into the spinal canal (retropulsed). Burst fractures **(Figure 10.8)**, may involve one or more vertebrae, and are commonly associated with neurological deficits due to the fragments being retropulsed into the spinal canal. This injury can occur from a motor vehicle crash or a fall.

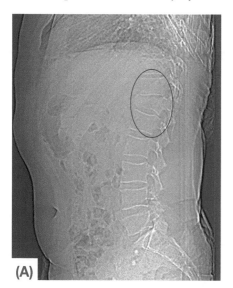

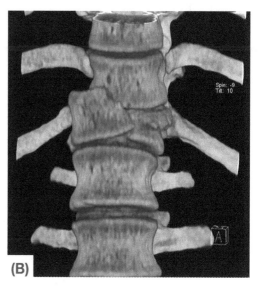

(A)   (B)

FIGURE 10.8 (A) Burst fracture; (B) burst fracture CT scan 3Dl reconstruction.
Source: Courtesy of Dr. Douglas W. Parrillo.

A chance fracture can occur from wearing a lap belt or when children are not properly restrained in a correct child safety seat during a motor vehicle crash. Chance fractures are transverse fractures through the vertebral body, pedicle, and spinal process. This fracture is most seen in the lower thoracic and upper lumbar spine and may be associated with intra-abdominal injury **(Figure 10.9)**.

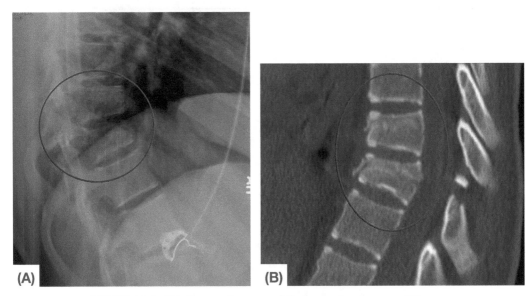

(A)   (B)

FIGURE 10.9 (A) Chance fracture; (B) chance fracture on CT scan.
Source: (A) Reprinted by permission of James Heilman, MD, Wikipedian, ER Department Head, East Kootenay Regional Hospital, Clinical Assistant Professor, Department of Emergency Medicine, University of British Columbia; (B) courtesy James Heilman, MD, https://en.wikipedia.org/wiki/Chance_fracture.

CONCLUSION

When evaluating the thoracic spine, it is important to make sure that there is proper alignment, bone integrity, and disc space. This can be evaluated on both the AP and lateral views. Although the thoracic spine is better protected than the cervical spine, it still has the potential for significant fracture and injury and may also co-occur with significant chest and abdominal organ involvement.

RESOURCES

Au-Yong, I., Au-Yong, A., & Broderick, N. (2010). *On-call x-rays made easy*. Churchill Livingstone, Elsevier.

Daffner, R. H. (2014). Musculoskeletal imaging. In D. H. Daffner & M. S. Hartman (Eds.), *Clinical radiology: The essentials* (4th ed., pp. 482–533). Wolters Kluwer/Lippincott Williams & Wilkins.

Gaensler, E. H. L., Purcell, D. D., & Watanabe, A. T. (2018). Spine imaging. In W. E. Brant & C. A. Helms (Eds.), *Fundamentals of diagnostic radiology* (5th ed., pp. 314–323). Wolters Kluwer/Lippincott Williams & Wilkins.

Herring, W. (2016). *Learning radiology: Recovering the basics* (3rd ed., pp. 266–278). Elsevier.

Kuntz, A. F., Lai, W. S., Norton, P. T., Yao, L. L., & Gay, S. B. (n.d.). *Skeletal trauma.* https://introductiontoradiology.net/courses/rad/ext/

MacLeod, T. D., Auyeung, S., & Lazaro, R. T. (2020). Radiologic evaluation of the thoracic spine, sternum, and ribs. In McKinnis (Ed.). *Fundamentals of musculoskeletal imaging* (5th ed.). F. A. Davis.

CHAPTER 11

Basic Interpretation of Lumbar Spine Radiographs

There are many similarities between the thoracic and lumbar spines. They are both better protected than the cervical spine, and as a result, require significant force to cause injury. As with thoracic spine injuries, lumbar spine injuries are often associated with injuries to the abdomen, pelvis, and pelvic structures. Acute back pain can result from either fracture, sprain, or strain, or be caused by degenerative changes, overuse injuries, infection, or a herniated nucleus pulposus (HNP) or disc.

NORMAL

When evaluating the lumbar spine, obtain an anterior–posterior (AP) and lateral view **(Figure 11.1)**. Lumbar spine images should include the upper level of T10 if traumatic injury is suspected. Approximately two thirds of lumbar injuries occur at the level of T12 to L2, which is why imaging T10 and T11 is necessary.

While evaluating the AP and lateral views of the lumbar spine, carefully inspect the vertebral bodies, spinous and transverse processes, and pedicles on the AP view. On the lateral view, examine the inferior articular and superior articular processes. These areas are shown in **Figure 11.2**.

The vertebral bodies of the lumbar region will increase slightly in height as you scan downward toward the sacrum. The vertebral bodies should have smooth margins and be in full alignment. The disc spaces also increase progressing toward the sacrum except for the disc space of L5–S1 which is slightly narrower than the disc space of L4–L5. As with any other radiograph, make sure that you are evaluating the entire image from left to right and from top to bottom.

A—Image adequacy should be ensured prior to interpretation as with any other radiograph. Evaluating *a*lignment begins with the spinal processes. They should be readily visible on the AP view from the base of the cervical spine through to T4 or T5 and then again at the lower end of the thoracic spine. Both the anterior and posterior margins of the vertebra should be in alignment on the lateral view.

B—The vertebral *b*one (body) should have uniform margins that are aligned with no interruption in the margins. The pedicles should be visualized on the lateral view without any disruptions along their borders. It is important to note that in the lateral view the first four vertebral bodies are not readily visible because they are obscured by the shoulder girdle, superimposed ribs, and lung markings.

C—There is no *c* when interpreting the thoracic spine.

D—The intervertebral *d*isc spaces should get progressively larger with progression toward the lumbar spine.

S—The paravertebral *s*oft tissue line may be visible and is considered normal. However, any enhancement and/or displacement of this line suggests swelling and an injury. See **Figure 11.3** for the ABCDs (adequacy and alignment, body, cartilage or joints, disc space, soft tissue) of the L-spine.

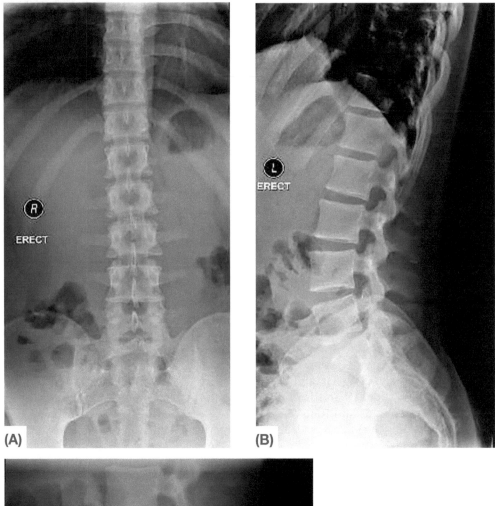

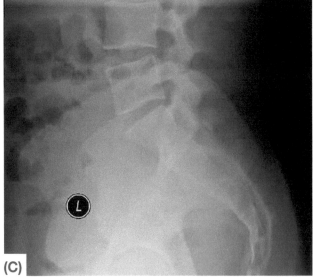

FIGURE 11.1 (A–C) Normal lumbar spine views.
Source: Radiograph.

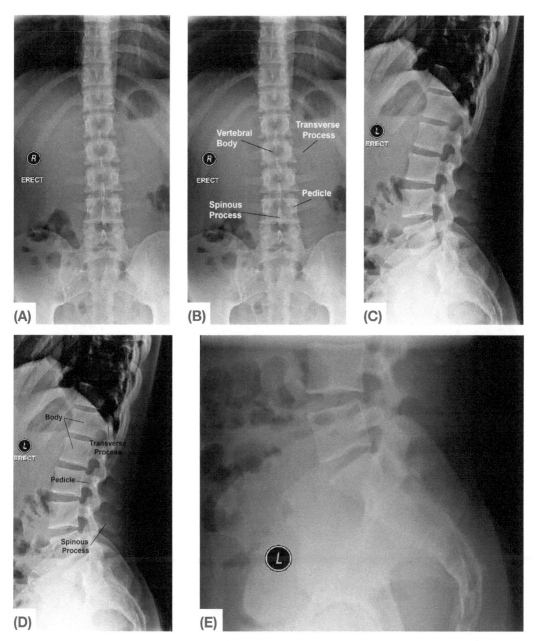

FIGURE 11.2 (A–E) Normal lumbar spine views with markings.
Source: Radiograph.

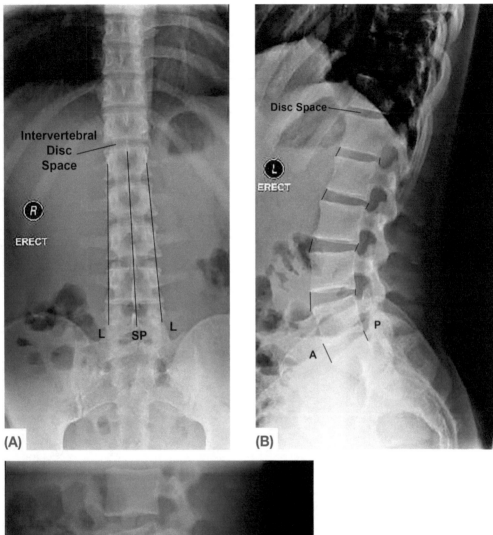

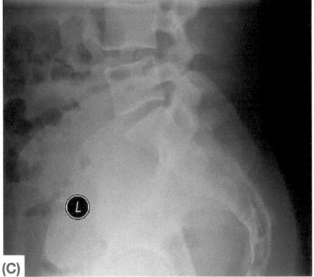

FIGURE 11.3 (A–C) Lumbar spine with disc spaces. A, anterior;
L, lateral; P, posterior; SP, spinal process.
Source: Radiopaediageneral@radiopaedia.org

ABNORMALITIES

Most injuries to the lumbar spine are similar to those found in the thoracic spine. These injuries, which include compression, wedge, and chance fractures, are typically found between the area of T12 and L2. Degenerative changes, such as spondylolysis, spondylolisthesis, and spinal stenosis, can also cause back pain and be identified on plain radiographs.

Spondylolysis is a break or defect of the pars interarticularis. It is thought to be a chronic condition that may be congenital or that develops post trauma after a fall to the buttocks during early childhood causing stress to the lumbar spine. This defect most often occurs at the level of L5 and can be identified on radiograph as a "Scottie dog" figure. This is best seen on an oblique view with the transverse process making up the nose, superior articular process making up the ear, contralateral superior articular process making up the tail, contralateral inferior articular process making up the rear leg, inferior articular process making up the front leg, the pars interarticularis making up the neck, and the pedicle making up the eye. The collar that appears around the neck of the dog is the defect. See **Figure 11.4** for the "Scottie dog" figure.

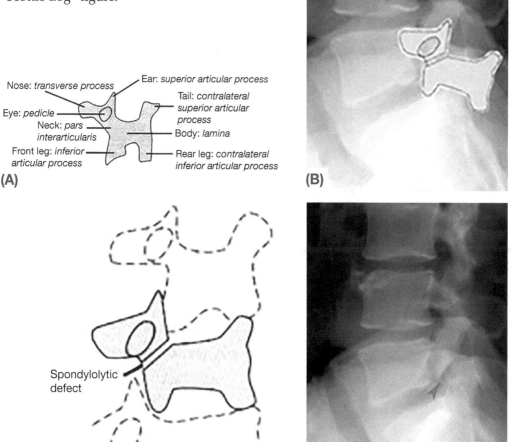

(A)

Nose: *transverse process*
Ear: *superior articular process*
Tail: *contralateral superior articular process*
Eye: *pedicle*
Neck: *pars interarticularis*
Body: *lamina*
Front leg: *inferior articular process*
Rear leg: *contralateral inferior articular process*

(B)

(C)

Spondylolytic defect

(D)

FIGURE 11.4 (A,B) Scottie dog model of lumbar spine; (C, D) spondylolysis.
Source: University of Virginia. Permission granted by the University of Virginia Department of Radiology and Medical Imaging.

Spondylolisthesis (Figure 11.5) occurs if there is bilateral spondylolysis with shifting of the vertebral body forward. This most commonly occurs at the level of L4–L5 and L5–S1. There are five grades of spondylolisthesis based on the percentage of shifting.

- Grade I   = ≤25%
- Grade II   = 25–50%
- Grade III = 50–75%

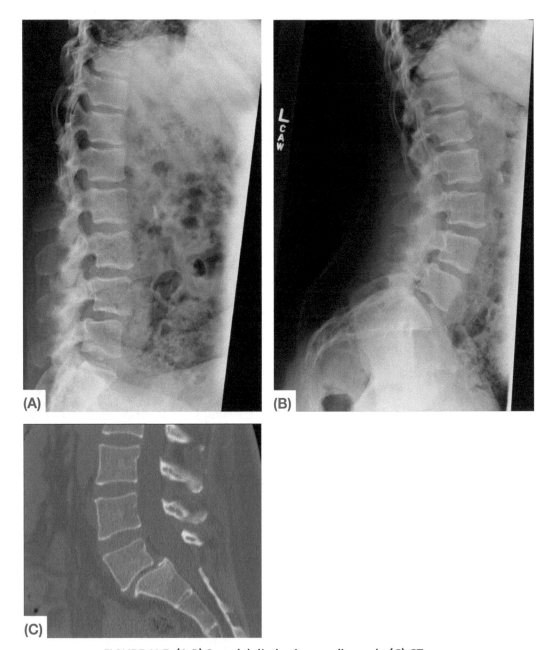

FIGURE 11.5 (A,B) Spondylolisthesis on radiograph; (C) CT scan.
Source: (A,B) Courtesy of Dr. Douglas W. Parrillo; (C) courtesy of Dr David Cuete, Radiopaedia.org, rID: 23567 (https://radiopaedia.org/articles/spondylolisthesis-1).

- Grade IV = 75–100%
- Grade V   = Complete displacement

If severe, there can be neural foraminal stenosis and impingement of the nerve roots in the central spinal canal. More commonly, spondylolisthesis is caused by degenerative facet changes.

Degenerative changes and stenosis can be visualized as bone spurring and loss of vertebral and intravertebral disc height. The degree of bone spurring and sclerotic changes can lead to fusion of the vertebrae. See **Figure 11.6** to visualize degenerative changes along the lumbar spine.

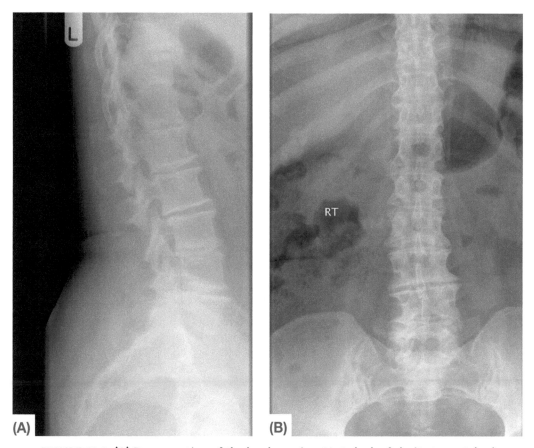

(A)   (B)

FIGURE 11.6 (A) Degeneration of the lumbar spine. Note lack of clarity to vertebral bodies and development of osteophytes; (B) degeneration of the lumbar spine. Note loss of vertebral body shape.
Source: Courtesy of Dr. Douglas W. Parrillo.

Vertical compression fractures can cause loss of height to the vertebral body in a crushing manner. See **Figure 11.7**, which shows a compression fracture. The severity of a compression fracture of the lumbar spine varies. Additionally, there is a natural tapering of the anterior lumbar vertebral body, which should not be confused with a compression fracture where there is loss of height as well as disruption of the posterior cortical line. Compression fractures are more common in women than men and may occur secondary to osteoporosis with minimal force. They most frequently occur in the upper lumbar

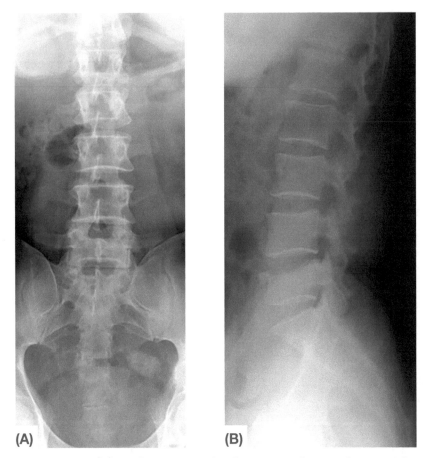

(A)   (B)

FIGURE 11.7 (A) Lumbar compression fracture on the anterior–posterior
and (B) lateral view. Note the loss of vertebral height on both views and
the malalignment of L4, L5, S1 on the lateral view. There is also a bone
fragment visualized in the lateral view.
Source: University of Virginia. Permission granted by the University of Virginia
Department of Radiology and Medical Imaging.

region and at the thoraco–lumbar junction specifically. Anterior wedge fractures may also
be identified and are more common at the thoraco–lumbar junction. Further evaluation
may be required with CT scan or MRI to identify associated spinal canal injuries or if there
is a strong suspicionbased on the history and physical of a fracture that is not visible on
the plain radiograph.

Lumbar chance fractures, like thoracic chance fractures, can occur from wearing a
lap belt during a motor vehicle crash or may occur in children who are not restrained
in a weight-appropriate child restraint device. Chance fractures are transverse fractures
through the vertebral body, pedicle, and spinal process most seen in the lower thoracic and
upper lumbar spine (Figure 11.8). These fractures may be associated with intra-abdominal
injury.

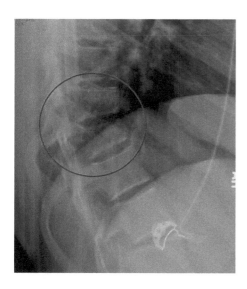

FIGURE 11.8 Chance fracture.
Source: Reprinted by permission of James Heilman, MD,
Wikipedian, ER Department Head, East Kootenay Regional
Hospital, Clinical Assistant Professor, Department of
Emergency Medicine, University of British Columbia.

Since traumatic injuries can cause fractures to the vertebral body, the pedicle, as well
as the spinous and transverse processes, it is important to evaluate all bony margins at
all levels of the lower thoracic, lumbar, and sacrum. Evaluation of the lower ribs as well
as the sacrum is imperative to ensure there are no fractures to any bony structures. See
Figure 11.9 for various L-spine fractures.

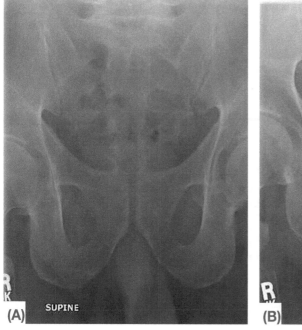
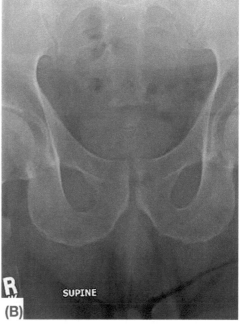

FIGURE 11.9 (A–D) Coccyx fracture.

(continued)

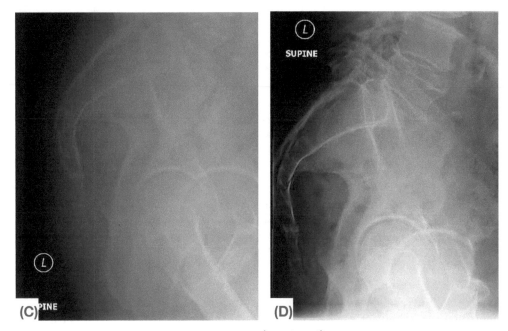

FIGURE 11.9 (*continued*)
Source: Courtesy of Dr. Douglas W. Parrillo.

CONCLUSION

Fractures and chronic changes of the lumbar spine can be easily identified on plain radiographs. However, if a fracture is suspected and not visualized on a plain radiograph, further study may be required for evaluation of occult fractures and soft tissue injuries. Overlying bowel contents and gas can further obscure structures of the lumbar spine or suggest a fracture line. When present, either repeat the image or follow up with a CT scan to rule out a fracture.

RESOURCES

Au-Yong, I., Au-Yong, A., & Broderick, N. (2010). *On-call x-rays made easy*. Churchill Livingstone, Elsevier.

Daffner, R. H. (2014). Musculoskeletal imaging. In D. H. Daffner & M. S. Hartman (Eds.), *Clinical radiology: The essentials* (4th ed., pp. 482–533). Wolters Kluwer/Lippincott Williams & Wilkins.

Gaensler, E. H. L., Purcell, D. D., & Watanabe, A. T. (2018). Spine imaging. In W. E. Brant & C. A. Helms (Eds.), *Fundamentals of diagnostic radiology* (5th ed., pp. 314–323). Wolters Kluwer/Lippincott Williams & Wilkins.

Herring, W. (2016). *Learning radiology: Recognizing the basics* (3rd ed., pp. 266–278). Elsevier.

Kuntz, A. F., Lai, W. S., Norton, P. T., Yao, L. L., & Gay, S. B. (n.d.). *Skeletal trauma*. https:// introductiontoradiology.net/courses/rad/ext/

MacLeod, T. D., Auyeung, S., & Lazaro, R. T. (2020) Radiologic evaluation of the lumbosacral spine and sacroiliac joints. In McKinnis (Ed.). *Fundamentals of musculoskeletal imaging* (5th ed.). F. A. Davis.

INDEX

Note: Page numbers in italics denote figures. Page numbers in bold denote tables.